Rey's of Sunshine

A Mother's Love Story

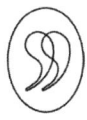

Rey's of Sunshine
A Mother's Love Story

NAVI SYAN GHATAORE

StoryTerrace

Text Navneet Ghataore

Copyright © Navi Syan Ghataore

First print August 2022

StoryTerrace

www.StoryTerrace.com

To my dearest, most precious possession Réyan, Words cannot express my boundless gratitude for you.

Thank you for giving me a purpose for waking up each day – you really are the best chapter of my life and the biggest inspiration. Today, tomorrow and always.

*Your biggest fan,
Mama*

CONTENTS

PROLOGUE — 9

CHAPTER 1: THAT MOMENT... — 15

CHAPTER 2: FINDING OUR VOICES — 23

CHAPTER 3: BROKEN CRAYONS STILL COLOUR... — 43

CHAPTER 4: RÉYAN'S DAY — 51

CHAPTER 5: THE 50-THOUSAND-POUND GAMBLE — 67

CHAPTER 6: SUNFLOWER BOY — 77

PROLOGUE

'Please tell me that's not Réyan's brain scan.'

Harnish and I are sitting in the consultant's office with nine-month-old Réyan. There are two pictures of a brain scan backlit on the monitor above us.

'I'm sorry to say it is,' says the doctor. I burst into tears.

'What's the matter?' says Harnish, looking from me to the scan and back again.

The black, white and grey patches depicted on brain scans are difficult to interpret, but as a Clinical Associate Practitioner I spent a lot of time working with stroke patients, so I could read them.

And at that moment, this one was a bit of a horror story. Réyan had a hypoxic brain injury. His brain had been severely damaged by a lack of oxygen, with a particularly catastrophic effect on the areas dealing with communication. The damage would also mean significant developmental delays and problems with movement and coordination. This sort of injury is usually classified under the term 'cerebral palsy', although every brain, and thus every person, will be affected differently.

We were told Réyan would never talk or walk, or even eat normally. Eye contact would be a big ask and might not ever be achieved. We were set up with a physiotherapy appointment at which they produced a wheelchair – a horrible metal contraption to my traumatised eyes, almost like something you'd find in a torture chamber. We were told our child would spend at least 12 hours a day strapped into this chair for the whole of his childhood. A tube would be inserted into his nose or stomach, and he'd get his nutrients via this: endless reconstituted sachets – but never having the pleasure of actually tasting a meal or the sensation of a sweet treat melting in his mouth.

I refused to accept any of this, and – spoiler alert! – this is not where we are today.

Today, Réyan is my sunflower boy. He needs a few sticks to hold him up – a bit more support than some of the other 'flowers' – but he's going to grow tall and strong and beautiful. He takes steps and gets around under his own steam using a walker. He might not speak, but he uses his voice and sign language to make himself understood, and we have full-on conversations. He eats with us at the table, either at home or in restaurants, and loves our regular trips to posh hotels for afternoon tea.

Most wonderfully to me, he has a smile as wide as a sunflower, and this puts a smile on my face every time I see him. He really is my Réy of sunshine.

Now, not accepting the life and the future the doctors and other medical professionals predicted for Réyan is vastly different from not accepting Réyan. I totally accept him, just the way he is. I would not change a hair on his head for all the world, but I would change the world for him.

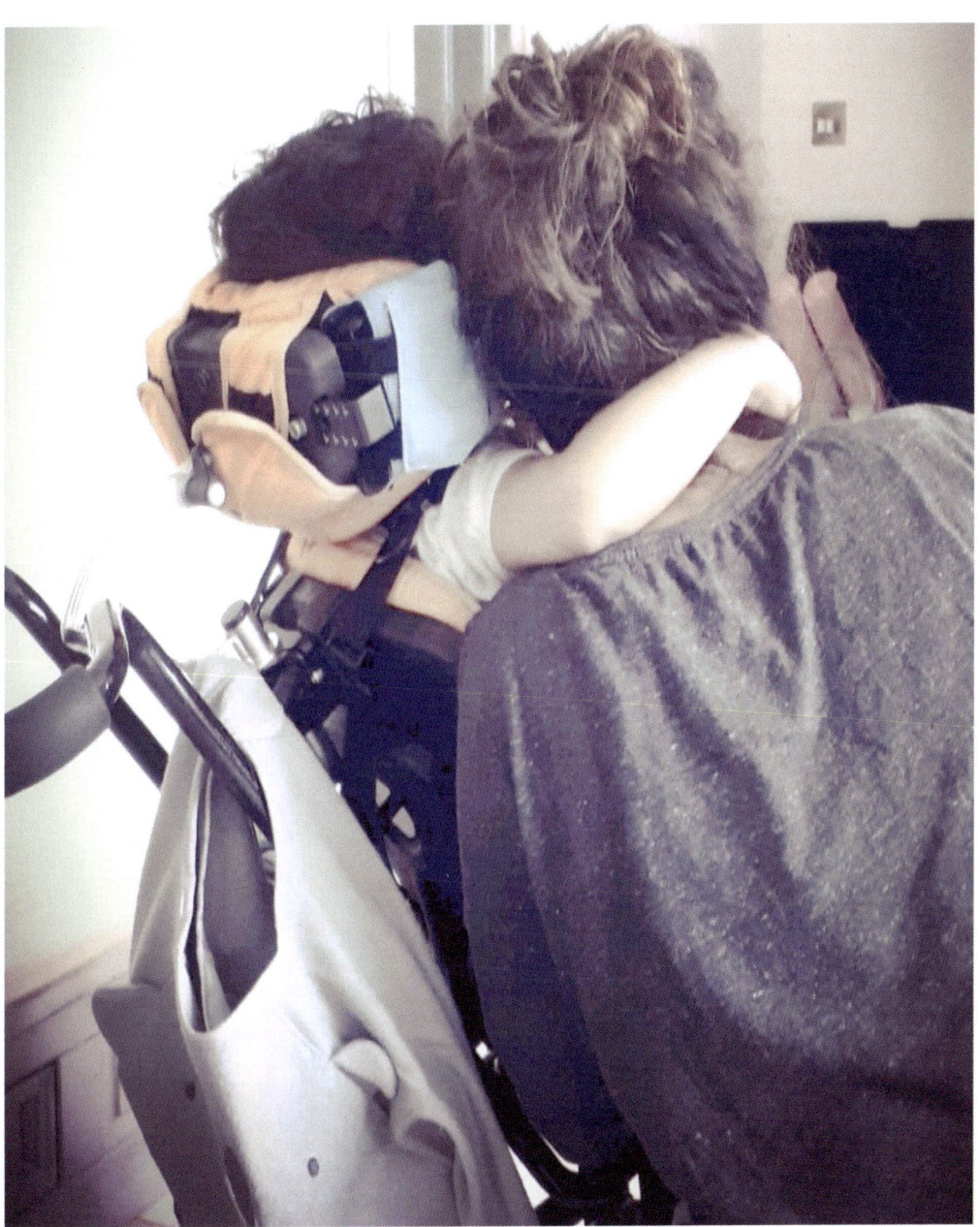

When you are the parents of a special needs child, life can be full of questions and suggestions. We sometimes feel bombarded by the curiosity of others, most of it well-meant, of course, but it can be overwhelming. There is also more than enough 'advice' to last a lifetime. That's why – although I hope people find this book helpful, possibly even inspiring, and definitely full of heart, whatever else it is – it is not an advice book. It's just a story about our family, our ups and downs, and how we've made things work. As my mum always says, 'Listen to everybody, and then do what you want.'

So, hopefully, this book will resonate if you are on a similar journey to us. But I also want it to reach further and perhaps open up our world a bit more, both to my fellow medical professionals and anyone who has a differently-abled child in their life or is just interested in a different perspective.

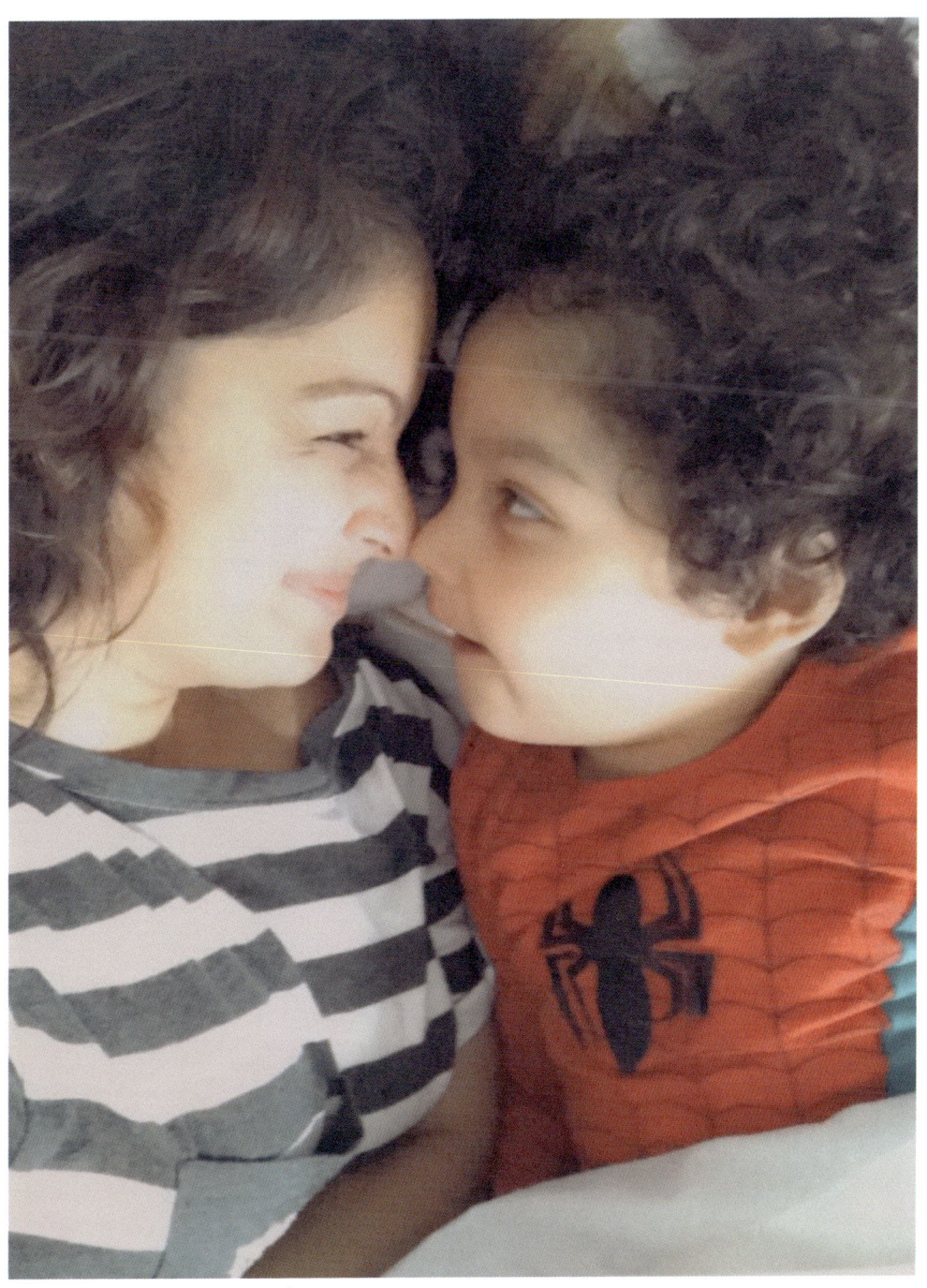

I got you baby

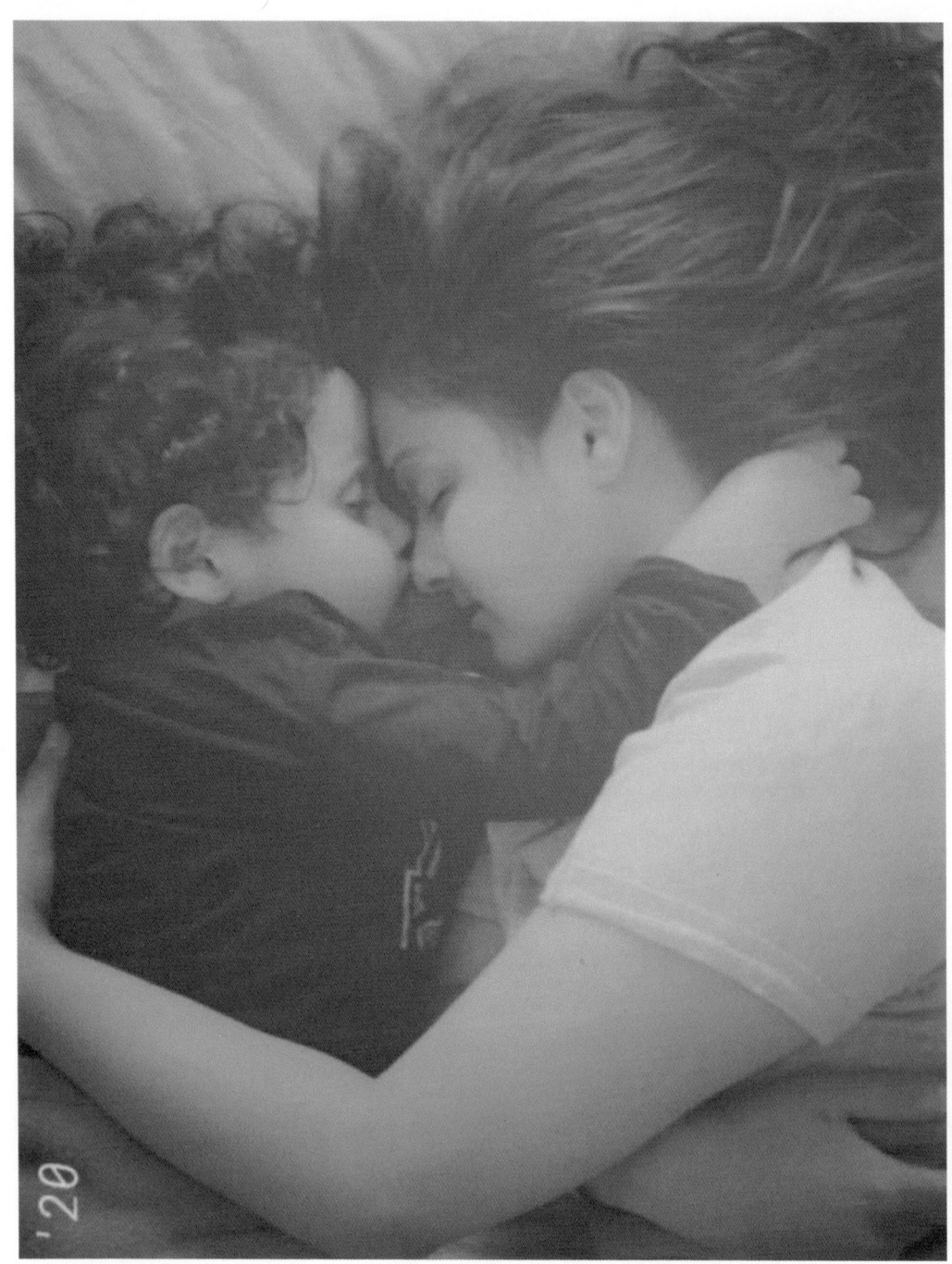

Safe with you

CHAPTER 1: THAT MOMENT...

I'm in hospital, attached to wires and tubes and surrounded by machinery. My heart beats at double speed, and my saturations are dropping. My oxygen level dips to 50. Beepers and buzzers go off all around. Doctors and nurses run around frantically, trying everything to get me stable.

Suddenly, the noise and the chaos fade into the background, almost as if I'm underwater or time has gone into slow motion, because there he is, a tiny bundle: my boy.

'It's me, Réyan! It's Mama!' I shout – although it's probably a barely audible croak. 'Look at me! I'm just over here!'

I lift a hand to wave and manage to raise it just off the covers. *Réyan, please recognise me,* I think. *Please know I am here.*

My mum and Harnish take turns holding up baby Réyan on the other side of the glass. He is just two months old, and for half his life, I have been here in the intensive care ward. He doesn't seem to recognise me. I take my oxygen mask off so he can see me better. There is more shouting from the medical staff, and the mask is firmly re-attached. I just stare and stare at this tiny perfect baby I have created – so near to me and yet, so far beyond reach.

At that moment, something changed inside me, and I was hit by a double wave of overpowering maternal love and a new fierce determination.

I have to get out of here. I have to get better. I have to get back to my boy and look after him. He has to know me.

It's different for every mother, the moment when she truly bonds with her child. That was my moment.

I'd collapsed at home when Réyan was just two months old and was blue-lit into hospital. I had to be resuscitated twice, and it had been touch-and-go for a while. Now, the sepsis was under control; I was stable but still very weak and, despite the pain that at times even morphine couldn't dull, I had only one thought: *I have to get home.*

I've always been a bit of a homebody. I'm blessed with a very loving family. One of my happiest childhood memories is Friday night pizza. We went to the same place every week and ordered exactly the same food every time – Mum, Dad, me, my sister and my brother. We nearly always sat in the same seats, and we would just chat and laugh, and I felt I was absolutely basking in the love of my family.

My mum was and is a very big influence on me. She's very playful, and I love that this younger self still comes out, even today. Our growing up was all about 'laugh until you're crying'. I always wanted to be like her, and she and my dad continue to be hugely supportive. They arrived in this country separately and completely on their own, then met, married and made a great life here. I really admire what they've built together, and it was a great foundation for us kids. They have a lovely house, our lifelong family home, but it's not just material things like bricks and mortar – they taught us how important it is to put your child, or children, at the centre of your life, and above all else, listen to them – really hear what they're trying to tell you, and be sensitive to their needs. I feel blessed to have such parents, as well as a sister who is also a best friend, and my baby brother, who, from the first time I clapped eyes on him, no one could adore more than me.

My parents' core value of working hard, but not so hard you forget to live or forget to notice how good life is, has stayed with me. Even today, if we're having a lovely time, I say to my husband, Harnish, 'Let's take a breath. Isn't this a lovely feeling, a great moment we're having right now?' It makes you smile, and instantly the day feels warmer. I am very much a sunny-side-up sort of person.

Growing up wasn't all a bed of roses; I had periods of illness and spent time in and out of hospital due to a delayed diagnosis of type 1 diabetes. Back then, for diabetes, it was isolation, masks and aprons – the whole lot. It was such a tough time. At school, some children thought you could 'catch' diabetes, so I also had to cope with a bit of bullying and also thought they would die coming close to me as it sounds like dia-bet-ic .

I'm naturally a calm person and was always a very 'good' child. Mum could dress me up in something pretty, and I'd stay sitting where I was put and not get dirty. But my experiences in hospital as a child taught me patience. Little did I know how much I would need that in the years ahead!

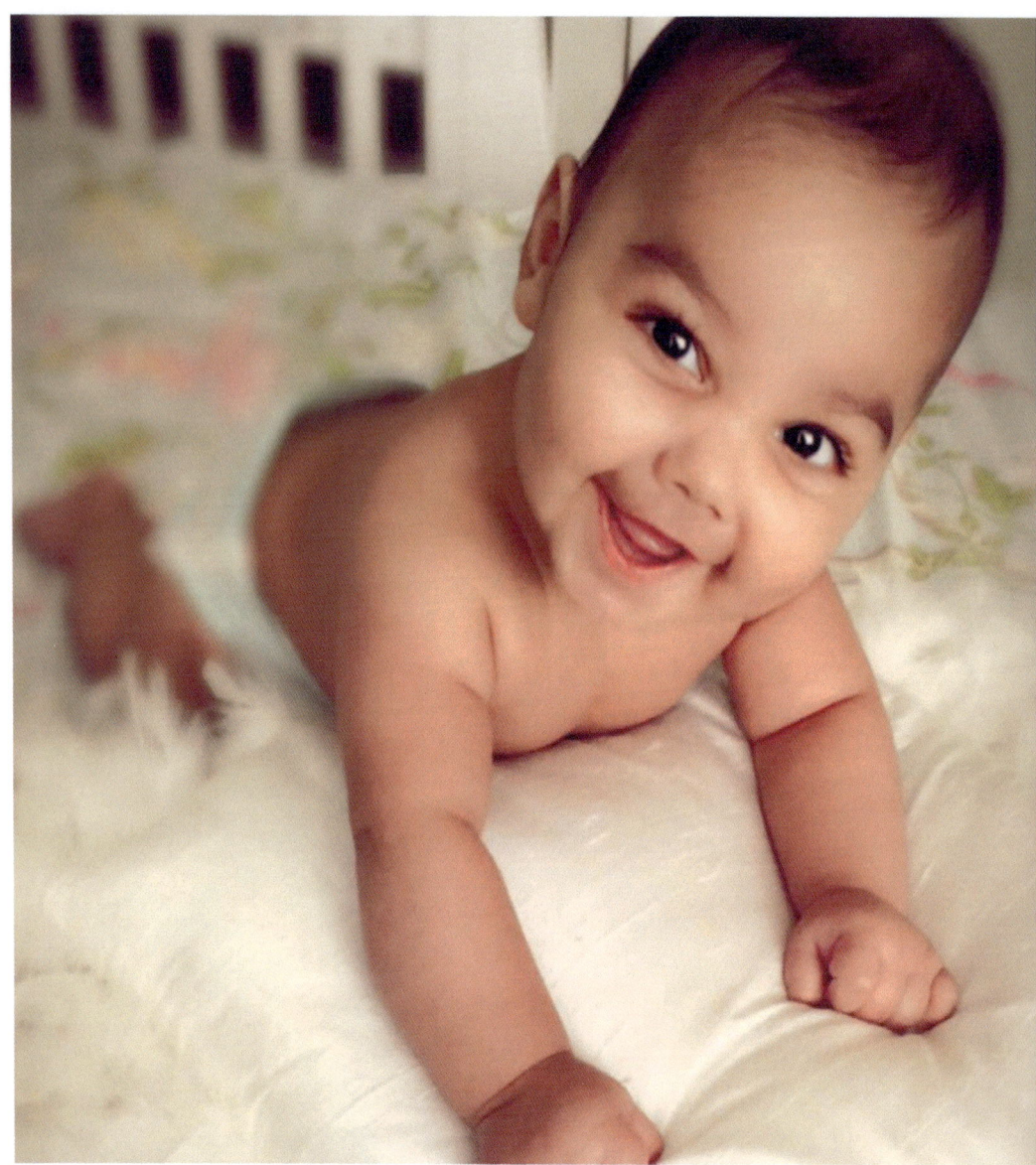

I've also always been very maternal, probably partly due to being the eldest and with quite a big age gap between myself and my younger brother. I know I've always had the ability to make people feel very secure and warm – it's something my family has always remarked upon. And if anyone's unwell, I love it! Not really, of course. I don't enjoy people feeling ill, but it's an opportunity for kisses and cuddles and making someone feel better.

So, I always knew I was going to go into health care – and I still absolutely love it. I worked a lot on stroke wards and progressed to become a clinical associate practitioner. I'd sometimes leave hours after my shift officially ended because a patient wanted to talk or needed something. I just couldn't leave if there was still anything I could do to help one of my patients! I found that if I was having a bad day but then went to work and managed to help someone, I would feel so much better. It's really helped me, and I'm proud to be living my life in the service of others.

I believe my background, upbringing and training, as well as my natural personality, gave me a toolbox of assets that equipped me exceptionally well for everything our little family has been through over the last five years. That's not to say it hasn't been hard. I had no idea, lying in that hospital bed looking at my gorgeous boy, that I was going to need every gram of patience, mental strength and creativity I possessed in the coming years. But I did know I had so much love, love unbounded, for that little scrap of life wrapped in his blanket. And that was the most important asset of all.

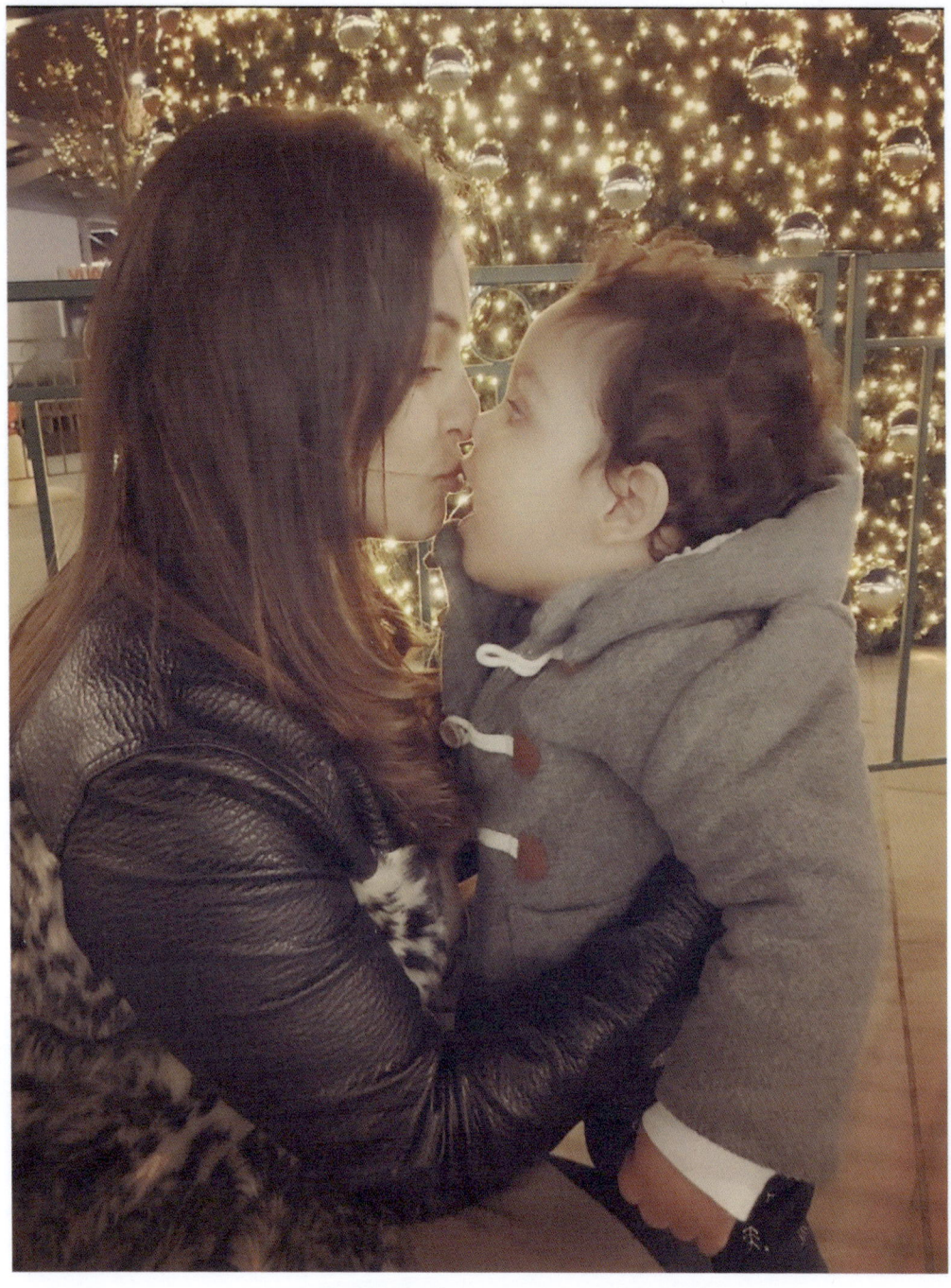

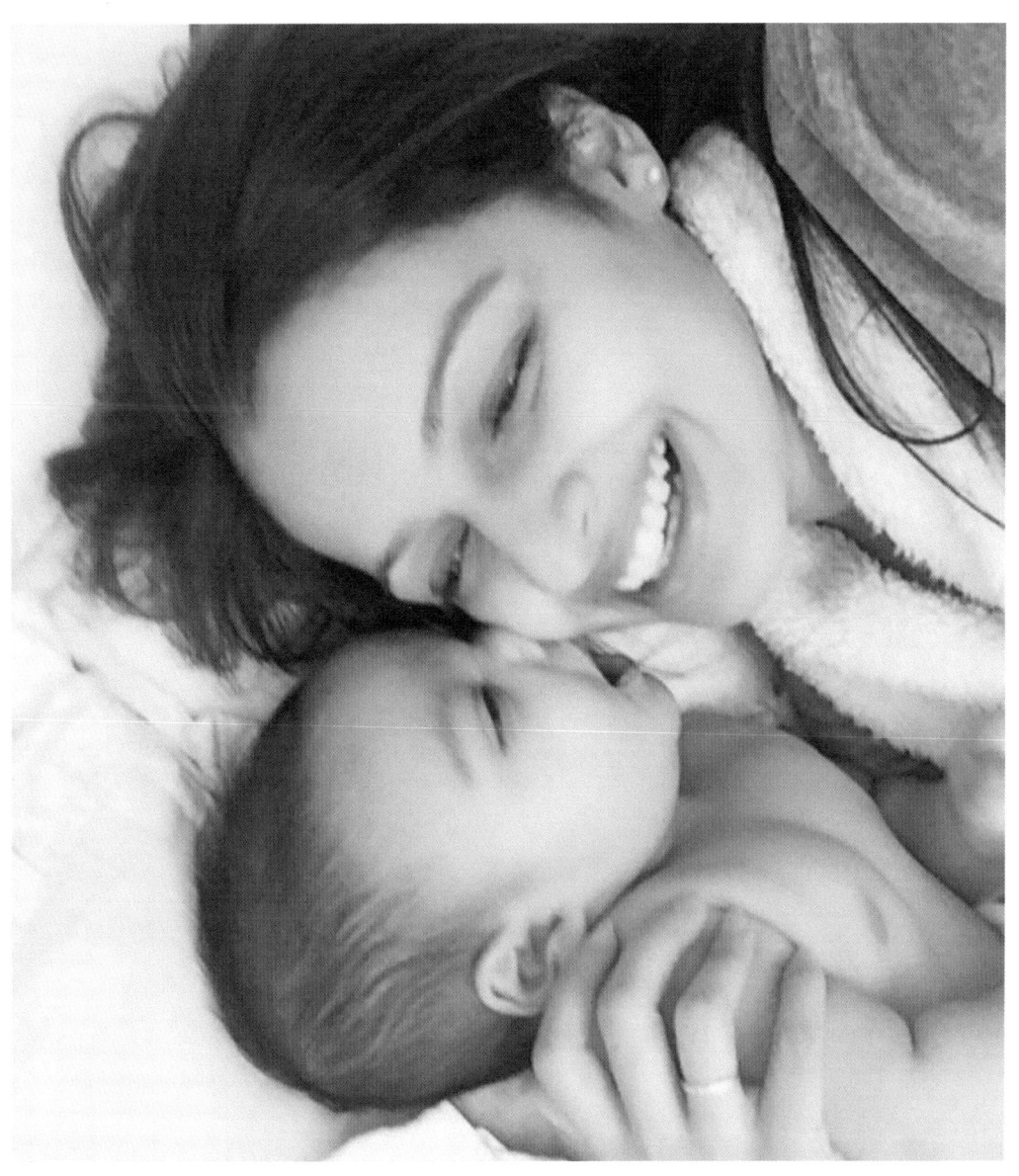

Mumma's precious soul

CHAPTER 2: FINDING OUR VOICES

When I came out of hospital, I started to think Réyan may have some developmental problems. He just wasn't hitting his milestones, and even more seriously, he was always choking at home. We were having to resuscitate him ourselves. I even taught Harnish how to do it in case Réyan choked when I wasn't there. I made repeated visits to A&E but was sent home with a metaphorical pat on the head and advice on holding him more upright while feeding. Or I was told the crackling I could hear in his chest was a chest infection, and we were given antibiotics. He had so many courses of antibiotics that he developed a resistance to them, and they stopped working so effectively. I was at my wit's end. I knew deep down something wasn't right, but it was difficult to fight the view of everyone around me that I was just an over-anxious first-time mother.

One day, I'd had enough. I put Réyan in his pram and set out for Great Ormond Street Hospital in Central London. We went to the private wing and had the brain scan I described in the opening of this book. I don't think I need to stress how devastating learning the results of that scan were for Harnish and me. But we picked ourselves up and forged ahead, trying to do everything we could for Réyan. We had to; there was no support or help, except from my wonderful family. I thank them every day for all they do for us.

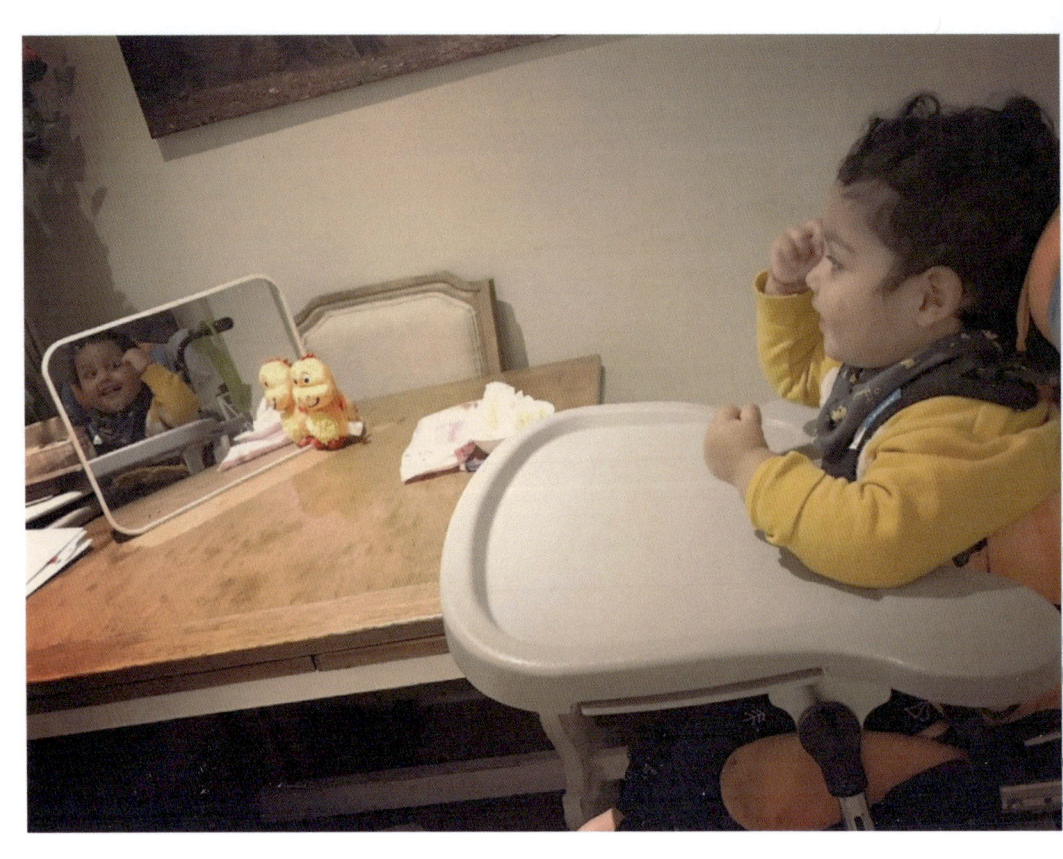

One of the first things was getting Réyan to eat and stop him choking. I started by giving him what was essentially thickened water – you can't choke on a drop. As with every obstacle that's come up during our last five years with Réyan, I find a way.

Other tricks that worked included smearing his favourite yoghurt onto the edge of a glass so he had to close his mouth to suck it off. If he can close his mouth, he won't drool so much he's exercising those muscles; he should be able to speak, and that's the train of thought the whole time.

I also put raspberries on the ends of each of his fingers too, once again, work many of his sensory skills. He had to concentrate and use all sorts of different muscles to eat them, he didn't like the sensation so he had to open his little fists which we couldn't get him to do, physios would suggest meds to minimise the spasticity but I thought we'll he can't use one hand as he's always got it in fists this way he will want to put his hand in his mouth to take off the raspberries -great way to feed himself, then he didn't like this sensation so he started to open his hand and then realised we did all of this without meds. but he never thought he was being taught – it was all a game!

There is a danger Réyan's life could become one long list of instructions. He learns differently than most people. Many of the things we take for granted, he has to be taught as individual steps. For instance, we just open a door, and a fully functioning toddler will learn that all as one. But with Réyan, it's, 'OK, let's turn the key, now lift the handle, push it back or forward.' It's a conscious effort rather than automatic. It's exhausting for him. I've always been very conscious of that and tried to rein back on the 'do this, do that' monologue and make everything as fun as possible. But also never rushing him, so there's never any pressure. Whatever is next will wait. It's so important I do everything around him very slowly so that he can do all the steps and be fully part of whatever activity is happening.

As Réyan progressed, Harnish and I decided to eat a soft diet for some time so he could see what we were eating. That produced a transformation – he wanted to eat what Mumma and Dada were having! He now loves food and eats so many different things, which is lovely for us as a family because Harnish and I are real foodies. Now, at five years old, he doesn't always eat exactly as we are eating. But, for instance, if we're going to a Japanese restaurant, I'll explain that to him and say we're all going to have to eat Japanese food. He's loves to explore new flavours and always willing to try. He understands the concept of chopsticks, although he can't use them. I have to do all that hard work, but he understands what's going on, and, vitally – he's part of the experience.

Sandwiches presented a bit of a problem, especially as I love afternoon tea. But we worked on it, slowly, slowly taking small bites, starting off with just butter but progressing to mayo and then cream cheese, purée veg and different types of flavours of bread. Nowadays, we love to go for afternoon tea together. We quite often treat ourselves to a trip to Hotels in London. It's not exactly a cheap option, but there's disabled parking nearby and the staff are brilliant. They really go the extra mile to make it a lovely experience for us.

Another place we really value is Piccolino in Virginia Water, Berkshire. We've been there so often that Réyan asks for a menu, and they take his order from him and don't talk over him. We ask them to over-boil the veg with the risotto – which must be torture for the chef! – but it means Réyan can eat it. Their whole attitude means we don't feel different; we're the same as any other family having a meal out, and it's wonderful. Another amazing place is Chennai express my god they love reyan and would to any length to help and keep us happy.

There are so many barriers for special needs children, and as parents, we are constantly clearing the way ahead, smoothing the path, but if someone does that for us once in a while, it's worth more than any amount of money.

When we go somewhere, we're often told they can't cater for Réyan, so I say, 'Do you have a potato? Yes? Great – mash that up. Do you have toast, a bit of cheese? Cheese toastie! Done!'

But I do want to stress that all this took a long, long time. We were left on our own as a family to cope in the early days. When he was a small baby, we were regularly resuscitating Réyan at home, so he was already under a lot of risk. My view was we couldn't put him any more at risk by trying to feed him. Gradually, he stopped choking so often, and by the time we were referred to physiotherapy and speech and language therapy, we had – by taking matters into our own hands – leapfrogged over where they were going to start with him.

Réyan's medical team still wanted him to be fed by tube, and I had a big battle because they really pushed for a peg feed. This would mean just reconstituted sachets of this or that for

Réyan. But by that time, he was already tasting foods, and if we'd stopped, he would have lost his mouth muscles and everything he'd gained. They advised us to wait, start it later, and said some kids begin at 10 years old.

Eventually, my persistence paid off, and we went away with the notes marked that we would 'risk feeding at home.' Being in healthcare I'm certainly not going to tell people to ignore their doctors. All I can say is that with a cautious approach and the unique knowledge everyone has of their own child, it can be done.

Since then, I've seen other parents struggling. They are often in a far worse situation than us just because they've done what the doctors told them to do. I feel bad when I share my stories. But there are some benefits to peg feeding, and some people get on with it great and are very happy with it. If it works for them, that's brilliant. My whole outlook is that not every child or every family is the same and that by trying to manage special needs children and squeeze them all into the same box, the medical professions do some of them a disservice. I just ask them to consider being more ambitious right from the start. I appreciate doctors want to cover their registration not get the parents hopes up but if you can't give us hope then don't take away the only chance they have, which is hope. I live in hope.

I remember one afternoon when I'd taken Réyan to a therapy centre, and there was another woman with a son who was about 10 years old. He had a very good oral intake, meaning his tongue and the way he swallowed was all working properly, much better than Réyan, and he could even drink with a straw, but he had a peg tube in. His mum got a bag out and prepared to give him a feed. Meanwhile, I had a bag of Wotsits for Réyan and was giving them to him one by one, telling him, 'Slowly now, let it disintegrate in your mouth.'

A slight diversion here: people are often surprised Réyan understands words like 'disintegrate', but why wouldn't he? If he can learn 'melt', he can learn its synonyms. It's just a question of using and repeating the words like you would with any child. There's so much more to Réyan – and other special needs children – than meets the eye.

Anyway, the mum at the centre was fascinated by this bag of Wotsits, and we got chatting. Her baby had been premature, so unlike Réyan, who was born at full term, she got support from day one. She'd followed what the doctors recommended and gone with the peg tube. She was so impressed by what Réyan was doing that she wanted to try her son with a Wotsit there and then. But I said no, he might aspirate – breathe it in – and choke. I saw her again three weeks later. She hurried over to me and said, 'After I saw you, I couldn't sleep; I was thinking about Wotsits! So I tried one with him. I've never seen his arms and legs go up in the air like that before. He was so happy!'

Well, that was just the beginning; then came cream cheese sandwiches, mash and gravy. Wotsits were the start of everything! I can't begin to describe how delighted I was for them!

It's always worth talking to other parents and getting a second, or even a third, medical opinion. There's always something to learn, and there might be just one bit of information that helps. I try to remember no question is a silly question – if my question is not answered, I just need to ask it again or re-phrase it until I get what I need.

We know the first five years are absolutely crucial for children. It's when the brain is developing the most, and their bodies are extremely flexible and supple. It's always seemed strange to me that while all the experts stress that point for able-bodied preschoolers, the system wants the differently-abled to wait. It just doesn't make sense. Push all the effort into the first five years instead of offering one physio appointment every six months. These special children may surprise everyone and go far beyond the initial prognosis, developing in ways that can benefit them, their families and the hard-pressed NHS for years to come.

To give another example, when we finally got a physio appointment when he was 9/10 months, it became clear the therapist wasn't interested in us as individuals and didn't even know Réyan's diagnosis. Nevertheless, she produced this huge, heavy scary chair – the one I described at the beginning of the book. It looked like something you could be executed in rather than something that you would want to spend any time in. The physio said Réyan needed to spend 12 hours a day sitting in it. Réyan goes swimming, and I thought if he can kick his legs in the water, he can kick his legs on the floor, but she wasn't interested. She was only interested in getting us to accept the wheelchair. Our lives flashed before me in that moment. I got very upset. I just could bare that thought. Me and harnish just couldn't make any eye contact with each other as we knew we were getting emotional.

'I know it's hard to accept,' she said, looking me straight in the eye. 'But you have to accept it. You should know better than anybody, being a nurse.'

'How dare you tell me that as a mother!' I replied.

I'm usually such a quiet, mild person, but that afternoon I was like a lioness fighting for my son's future. The physio didn't like my attitude and I was escorted out of the room. Our relationship never fully recovered, and the way the NHS works meant she was our physiotherapist for years. She's now been promoted and was now working elsewhere and we have someone who is much more on our wavelength – which is good news for all of us I suppose!

Now, if instead of 'acceptance', what if the attitude was to encourage families, and everyone supporting special needs children, to keep them out of the wheelchair as much as possible? Wheelchairs cost a fortune, and there's the risk of bedsores and all sorts of difficulties. A shift in emphasis could help everyone.

Réyan's developing differently, and every year the difference gets wider. His hips are growing differently because he's not using them. And teeth, for example, if they're not used to bite, they'll get longer in the mouth and are more prone to tooth decay. There really needs to be a re-think – a shift from expediency and managing the child within the system to a completely child-focused approach that connects the dots for these children and produces the best possible outcomes for

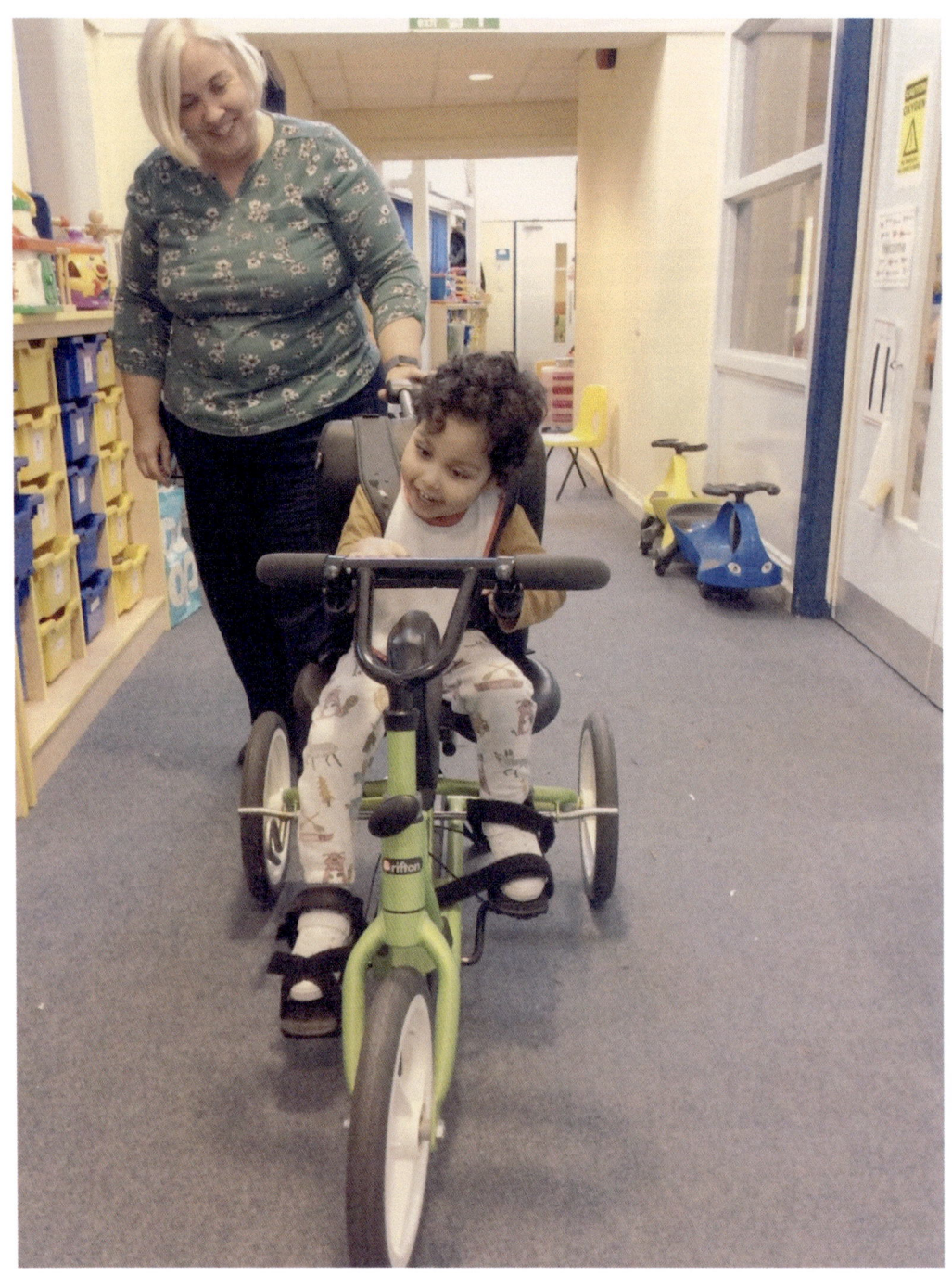

Catch me if you can

them – not what's most convenient. I dream of opening a centre for children like Réyan where I can put all my ideas into practice.

So, on to the next fight. I wanted Réyan to have a walker, but the NHS wouldn't give us one, as they said he wouldn't be able to use it properly. This is expensive equipment, and they are loathe to lend it out, so you really have to make a case for your child; the person I needed to convince was the same physio I'd already clashed with. But the wider point is that someone who sees Réyan once every six months – compared to us, his parents, who are with him all day every day and see improvements all the time – is the sole gatekeeper.

Réyan's school had a walker, and I begged them to let him have a go. He was so excited! Then he took his first steps! The teachers, all the staff, were running to see him.

'Oh my God, he's taking steps!' I shouted; Both me and harnish was in floods. It was an immensely emotional moment.

I sent videos to the physio, but her view was, 'That is not a good range of movement. Yes, he's taking steps, but he's not doing it correctly or using the walker correctly. It could damage his hips.'

My argument was, I appreciate what you're saying, but can we still try? The ball of the hip can fall out of place if it's not moving correctly, but the same can happen if it's not used at all. There's no muscle to support the socket. At least with the walker that area is being exercised, there are some muscles being developed in his bottom and the movement is good for

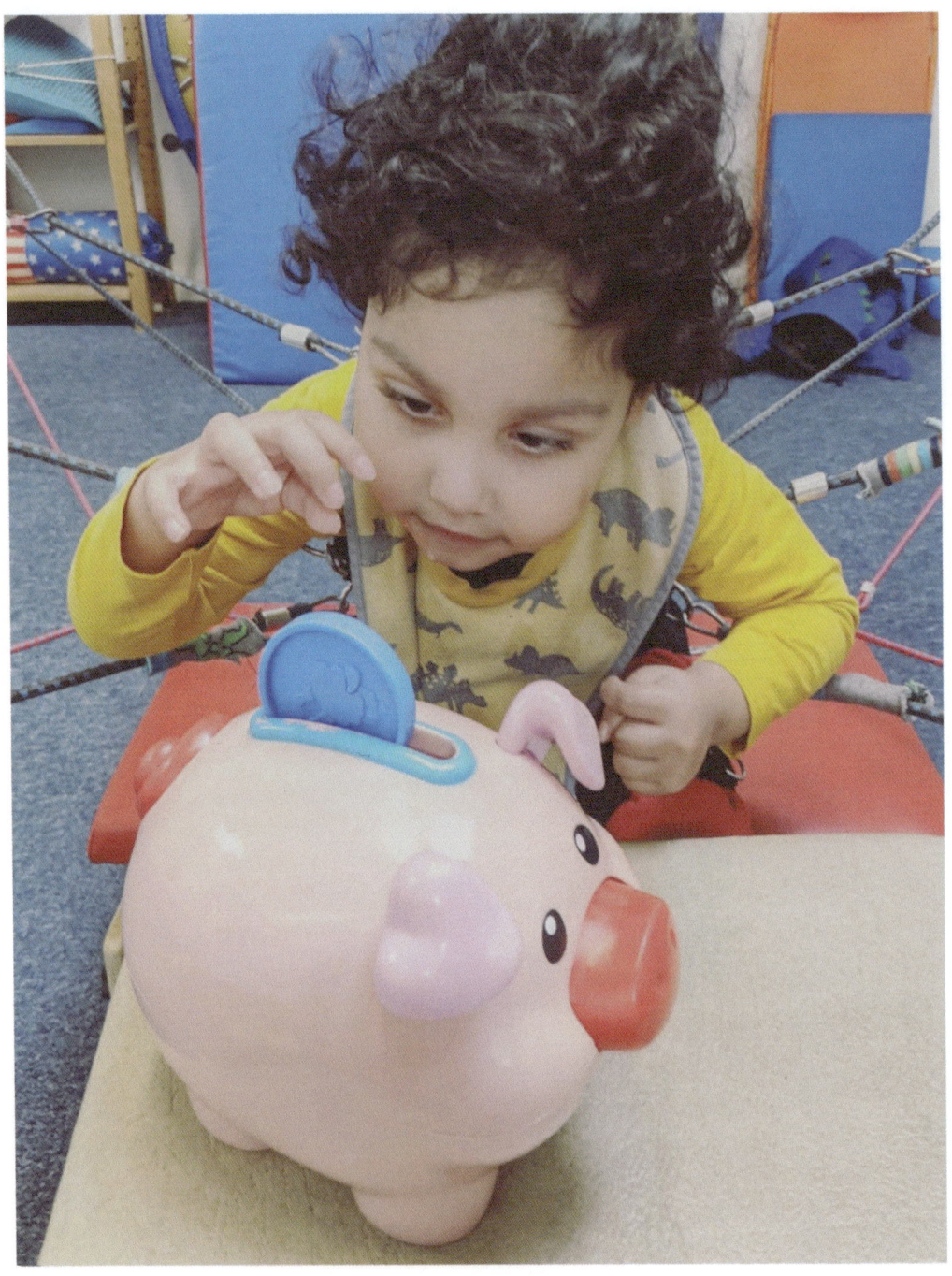

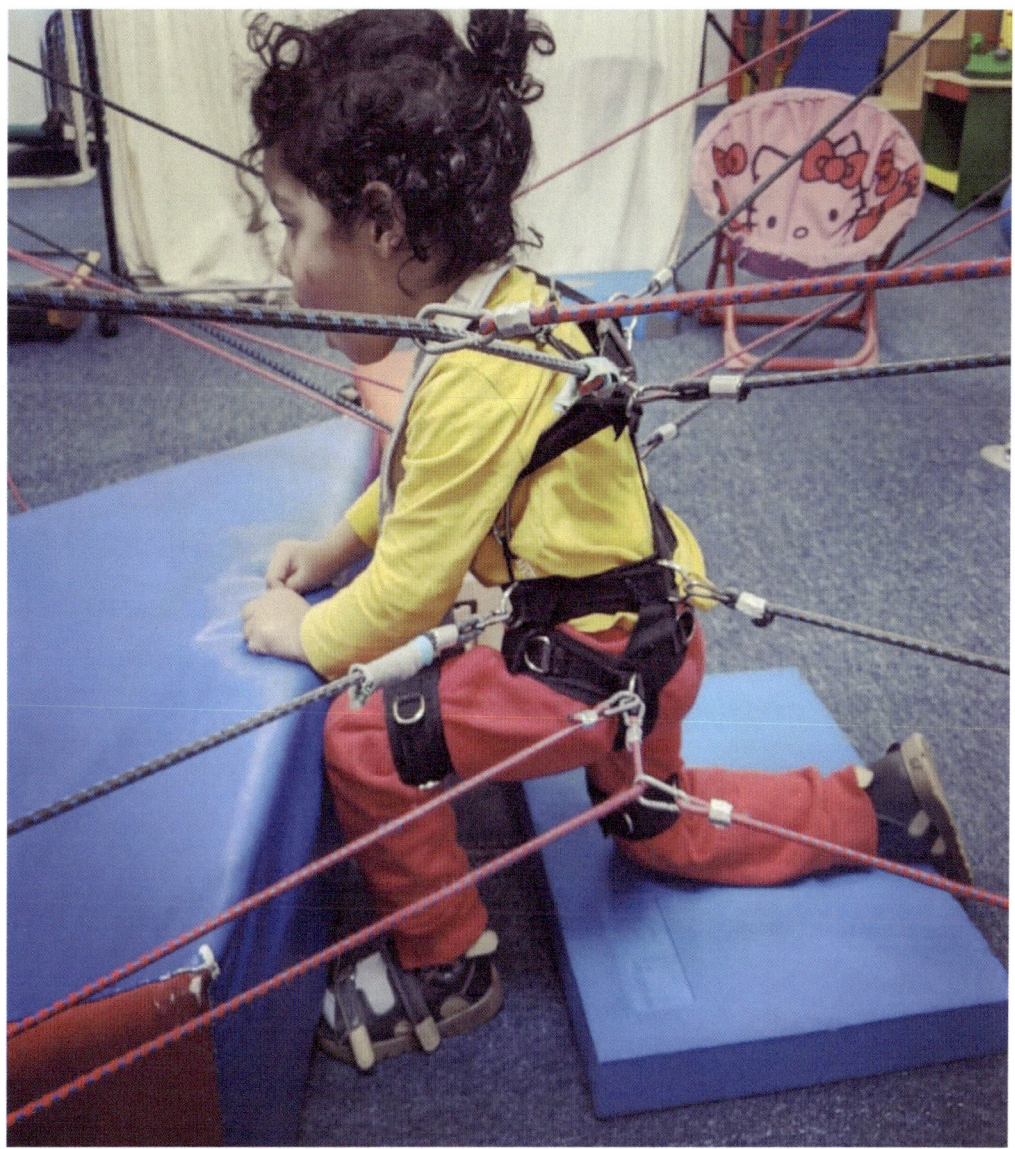

elasticity and stretching, which all helps with his spasticity. I don't care if his range of movement isn't quite right – we can work on that. I think they've got more of a chance if a child can see and understand what movement means and what walking feels like. It helps with motivation and makes them more determined. Above all, the walker gives Réyan precious independence.

In the end, after fighting and fighting and making my argument so many times, we got the walker – and it's changed our lives! Réyan loves it, and he really wants to walk correctly. I show him in the mirror and say, in the gentlest, most conversational way, 'Look at your foot; look at Mama's foot. Are they the same? No!' and he says, 'Ooh, ooh, ooh' and tries to do it properly. He tries so hard, and sometimes he can do it, and sometimes he can't. But that's ok we try and try and try until we can. Hope takes us a long way. Once again.

I love the NHS – it's been my life – and of course, it's important to be respectful of medical opinion, but I've learnt not to take everything at face value. Most medical professionals are brilliant at their jobs and very dedicated, but like anywhere, there's the occasional one who's not as good or maybe not as interested.

Conversations with medical professionals about special needs children can be difficult for parents to navigate, even when those professionals are very good and committed. They are often nervous about giving false hope but instead give no hope – which is not helpful either. I never tell people I'm a medical professional at the outset; it's not until partway into the conversation I let on that I know what I'm talking about. If I say it at the beginning, the staff start treating me better, and that's not good. Every parent should be treated the same – because they're the ones who know their children best.

If any medical professionals read this book, I'd love them to take away this message: please just listen. Not every child is the same – even two children with the same brain scan may present differently. They're individuals. Please consider carefully how you word things and the possible impact on parents. Be less brutal. Be more ambitious for children with special needs. Try not to concentrate on the negatives. Acknowledge a change in a child if you see it – however small it may be – and also acknowledge the hard work of the parents that brought it about. Some parents want a bit of hope or live on hope – give them that hope if they want it. Parents aren't stupid; you can tell the truth and say what is likely but then also say, 'There's just a chance this might happen.' Think about, 'What if it doesn't work?' but also ask, 'What if it does?'

I've learnt how to become a lioness fighting for her child. It has not come naturally at all. I wish I didn't have to scream and shout and keep asking and asking and even threatening to take it further. All I know is that I know Réyan best, and I have to keep fighting for my son. I am his voice and he is my heart.

The next challenge after finding my voice was to make sure Réyan also had a voice. Now that he understands everything, I think it's good that he hears me sticking up for him – fighting for what's best for him. But he also has his own voice. He

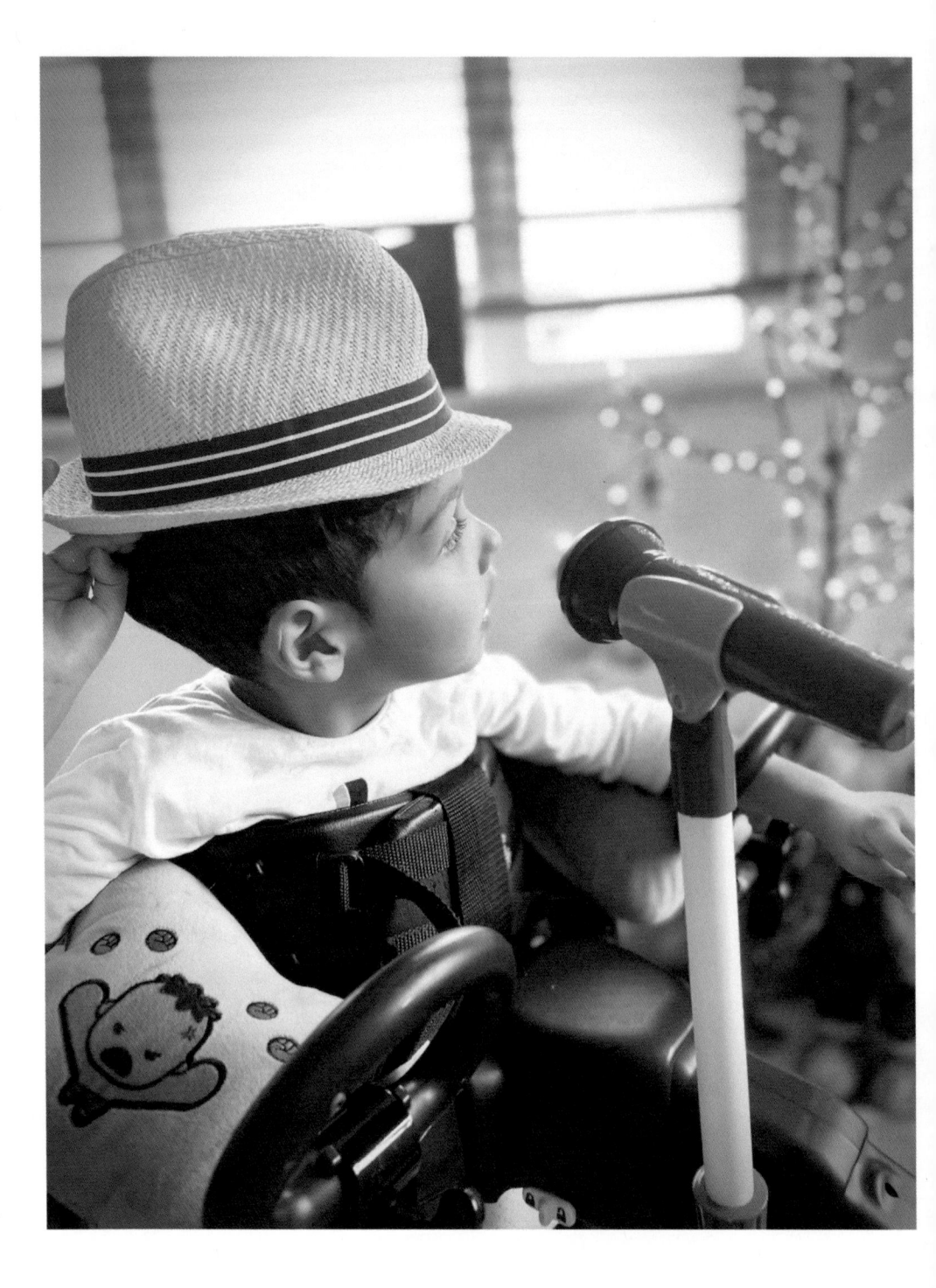

communicates all the time – how he's feeling, what he wants or needs, what he likes or finds funny. We have full-on conversations. A good ol' chinwag! As he gets older, it's important other people can hear him too.

All children need to learn the same things: colours, the common animals, numbers, etc. One of the first things we taught Réyan were the names of his body parts. We're always looking at things from his perspective – thinking about what is most useful and important for him. We also taught him how to express what he was feeling and put a name to those feelings. Everyone needs to feel they have a voice that is listened to, at least at home. If nowhere else, it's vital to know you have a voice there.

At one time, we had major problems with Réyan's medication and with his sleep. We'd tried everything, and he was on more and more drugs, which were having side effects – it was all spiralling in the wrong direction. Besides that, we all needed to get more sleep so we could function during the day.

We kept talking about the body with Réyan, and I put up a poster of a man and then cut up another one, so he could stick pictures in the right places. But we also tried to explain pain and give examples along the lines of 'happy – not hurt' and 'sad – it hurts.' Réyan was by now saying 'er' for yes and 'un' for no. Teaching him that was the best thing ever. I can do all the work with my questions, and he can just nod or shake.

The day he was able to communicate that his legs hurt at night was one of the best moments of my life! I went straight to his paediatrician to explain what I'd found out, and it resulted in him being able to take far fewer medications. He only takes one medication now, to help with his spasticity, and even that's a smaller dose than before. Réyan's bones are growing at a different speed to his muscles, and it causes pain in his legs and spasticity. He needs to stretch to loosen up in the morning, and the more he stretches, the better – so we do stretches throughout the day. Harnish regularly takes him swimming, which also really helps. The only thing we use now for sleep is a lovely mix of lavender and cherry blossom I found via Instagram.

Inevitably, as with any child, sometimes, how shall I put it . . . communication breaks down. If Réyan gets very fed up over something, I say calmly, 'You're shouting. Is Mama shouting? No. So why are you shouting? Are you having big feelings? That's fine; we all have big feelings sometimes. Let's try to sort this out, shall we?' I want him to know it's OK to not always be OK. Maybe he's got something important to say, but he's saying it differently. If a child's creating – don't go higher, go lower! Don't have an emotional tantrum yourself as an adult. You'll be more receptive if you press pause for that one moment, break off from broadcasting and see what you can receive. Otherwise, it can disintegrate into just a clash of energies. We can be so blocked by our own energies that we can't see what's going on in front of us.

A lot of people use 'time out' as a discipline method for children, but I actually think it works better as a strategy for parents! Think of a time when you can step away, maybe just an hour, and set an alarm if you need to. If you're particularly stressed, use it to cry, scream or let rip in some other way – look forward to it! I know I did sometimes! And then, when that hour is over, pull yourself back together, shake yourself off, do whatever's your thing, and you're a mum again.

Even five minutes can work wonders. If you are having a frenzied moment and just about to cry, go have a drink of water. Think of one thing: 'Why am I doing this?' – and the answer is because you love that person. Patience and perseverance goes a long way.

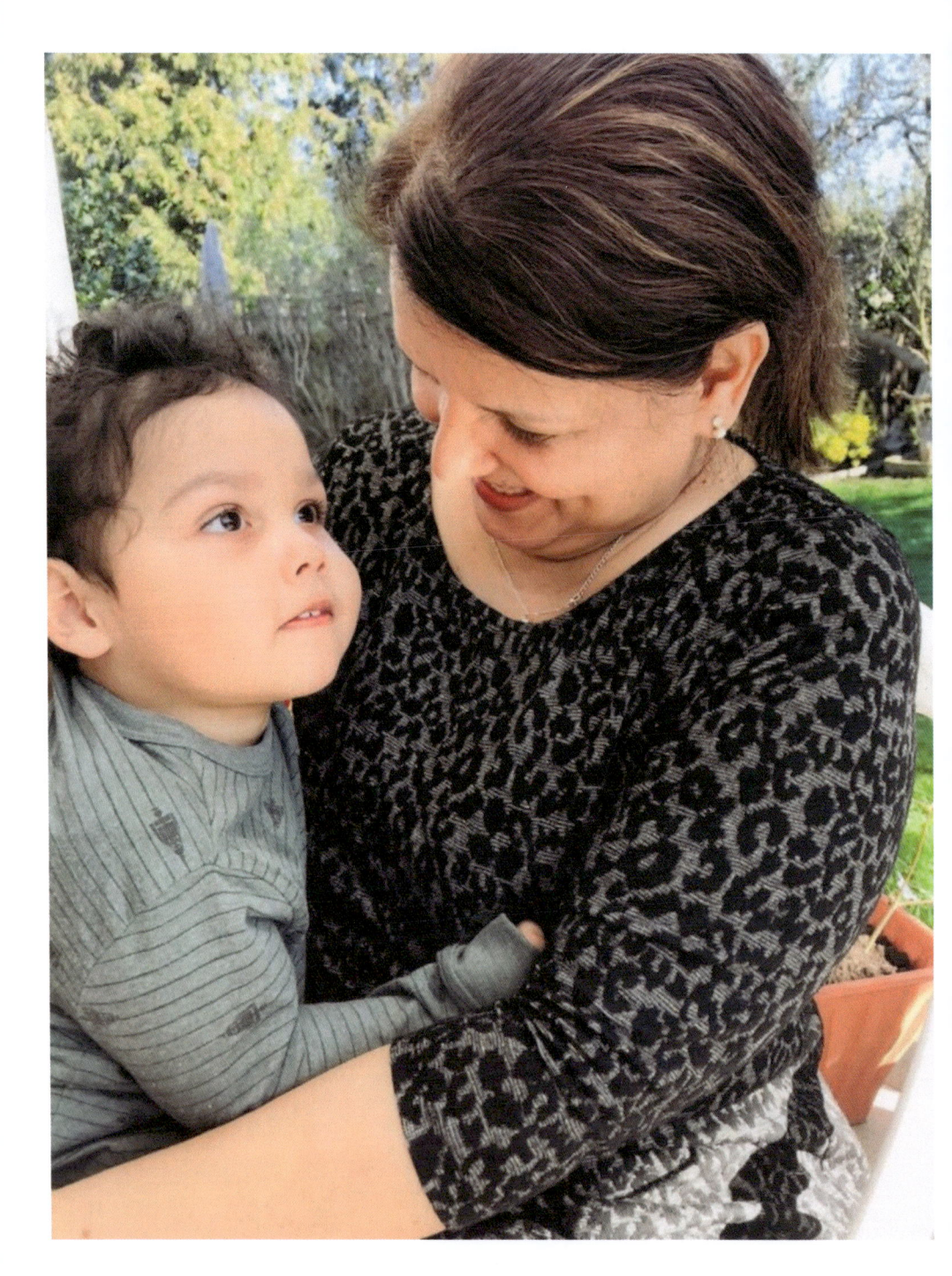

My baby's baby. Nani maa adores you

CHAPTER 3: BROKEN CRAYONS STILL COLOUR...

'Is he always going to be like this?'

'Will he ever get any better?'

'What's wrong with him?'

These are the 'smiling on my face, swearing in my head' questions. When you're the parent of a special needs child, it can sometimes feel as if it's raining questions. Believe me, I ask questions of myself all the time.

So, when someone asks if he's going to get better, sometimes I say, better?' I know what they're trying to say – they're asking if he's ever going to be normal. But this is my normal, and we're happy and content with it. To me, Réyan doesn't need to get 'better'. Like every other parent in the world, I think my child is perfect just being himself.

Other common questions include: 'Is he ever going to talk?', 'Are you going to have any more children?', 'Maybe if you had another child, you might not feel it so much?' and 'Maybe if you did a bit more of this or a bit less of that or flew to the moon or whatever, it might help. Have you tried that?'

Oh no, that's never occurred to us. We haven't spent hours, days, weeks trying everything, researching, planning and finding wells of patience we never thought we had. This is a variant on 'Oh, this or that drug is brilliant; you should try it. It really helped X or Y. They're doing great now.' OK, and you have a complete set of comparable medical records, do you? In order to prescribe for my child?

Obviously, I never say half these things out loud, and I never ever let Réyan see what I'm thinking or that I'm angry. But I do swear a lot in my head – or in the car or the shower. I never used to swear.

In the case of 'repeat offenders', as it were, I don't take Réyan to environments I'm not happy with or where I think the atmosphere is detrimental. I don't care who it is, and in our case, this does include a few family members who we now only see a couple of times a year when the event takes precedence and it's important we're there in order not to hurt other people's feelings. I am very happy with that. Réyan has helped me find my inner steel and not put up with things that can put my family's emotional stability – and this rock-solid unit we've built – in jeopardy. But it's hard work. It's not easy to be selfish.

The issue with one particular family member stems from before we even had a child. Harnish and I had been married for a number of years and were very happy, but we used to get nosey questions about when we were going to have children, and someone said, 'If you leave it too long, you'll have problems and you'll have a disabled child.'

The rational part of me understands there was no way they could have known what was going to happen with Réyan. But they've never apologised, and their attitude since has not always been helpful. Those words have played over and over in my head. I held them to my chest for a long time, and I am still so hurt by what was said. If I could ask for one thing, it would be to let go of that incident. Apart from anything else, it's so important I stay healthy in both mind and body. But I just can't forget it – words scar.

Things are easy to say but hard to take back. I wish people would just think before they come out with thoughtless comments. At my lowest, I felt almost as if a curse had been put over us, that we were paying the consequences for their mean words. Especially a family member said 'if you had left Reyan with us he would be doing so much better! Please move away before I say something I regret.

There have been other low moments. The true rock bottom was when our legal case against the hospital was rejected. It was a real hammer blow; I so wanted that compensation for equipment and treatments for Réyan. It also means that while we continue to field other people's questions, our most important question may never be answered – they can tell us what happened to Réyan but not how or why it happened, and there's not enough evidence to determine if any element of my care during pregnancy was responsible.

We've picked ourselves up and moved on, and I don't want sympathy, or judgement. There is a lot of sympathy, which is generally well-meaning – but we really don't need that! Empathy, yes, that's helpful, and I hope outlining some of our daily routines in this book will help people understand our challenges a bit more, but it's a bit disconcerting when people say, 'I *am* sorry' or 'Poor Réyan, poor boy.'

Réyan is certainly not a poor boy! He's surrounded by love, and he's happy every day. He is a lucky boy! And what exactly are they sorry about? I wish I could do more for Réyan. I want him to experience everything. But for Harnish and me, we are happy and we are fine.

The other phrases that wind me up are things like, 'I don't know how you do it' or 'You're doing so well' because they can sound a bit patronising. But I tell myself, 'This person is really just asking after us. I know they have a good heart. How they said it just went a bit wrong.' I have to be a bit forgiving, a bit accepting. People are trying their best.

I want people to understand our lives are not necessarily how they imagine them to be. My sister says, 'Why do you think you have to prove anything?' But it's not that; it's just that I'd like there to be a different narrative for once and open up our world for people, especially to convey the joy that Réyan brings to it. He's a delight.

We concentrate on – and are grateful for – everything that's positive. For instance, Réyan can't talk or walk, but his lip reading is amazing, his hearing is amazing and his sense of taste is much sharper than normal. So, although some things aren't working fully, others are much more powerful than is usual.

I'm sorry if some of the above sounds a bit angry, but none of us are saints – anger is fine every now and again! It can feel good to let it out. I know that people mostly mean well, and usually, it's water off a duck's back to me. But explaining things, especially things which are upsetting or emotionally triggering, over and over again to different people, can be exhausting. What's more, now he's older, Réyan's vocabulary is quite broad. It's not right that people talk over his head and assume because he can't speak, he can't understand either.

What is brilliant is when people are really sensitive and think about what specific help we might need. Or they don't ask – they just do. When people say, 'If you need anything, please let us know,' it's easy to worry that they don't really mean it. They probably are completely genuine and just don't know what to offer, but it's difficult to restart that conversation from cold and ask for a favour out of the blue.

We have a really good friend who doesn't ask, 'Do you need help?' He will just rock up at the door with food and say, 'Réyan's been poorly today, so the last thing you need is to cook. Here's dinner. I'm not stopping. It's on your doorstep.' And that's just wonderful.

We also had the chance to reciprocate when he and his partner were isolating during the pandemic – it was lovely to be able to pay them back for their kindness. That's also something important: please let us get involved! Sometimes people think, 'Best to leave them alone; they've got enough on their plate.' They are almost nervous of us. But we want to be treated like everyone else. Small things like this can make a huge difference.

Harnish and I also needed to learn lessons, and one of the most important was how to accept help. For instance, we didn't take any financial benefits for the first three years because we felt we were both working, we had a good standard of living, so

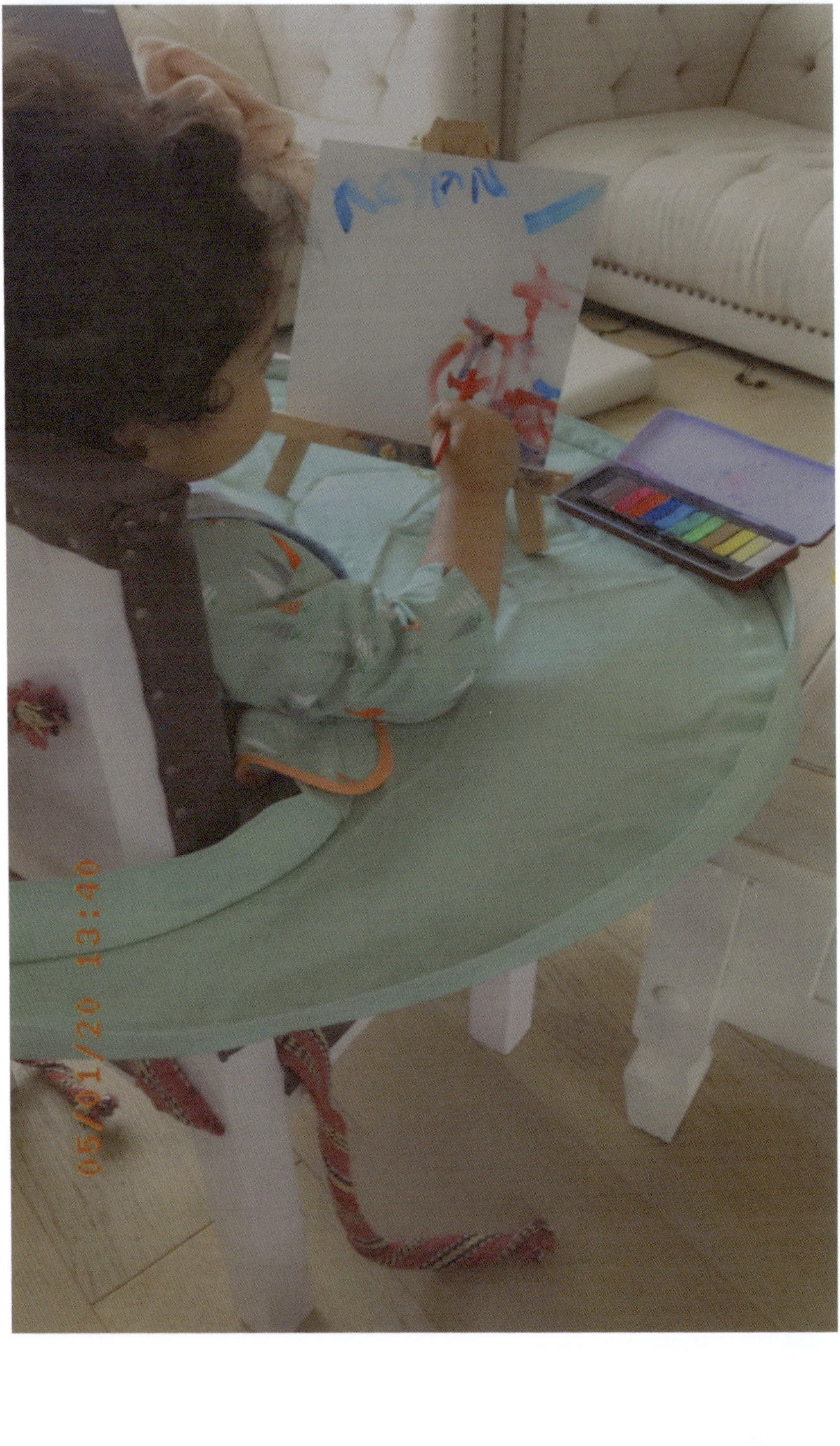

we didn't need it. We believed we should leave benefits for those in real need. We also thought it would only be natural that once the money started coming, we'd rely on it – then what if things change, and suddenly the rug is pulled from under us? You meet special people along the way who encourage you.

But after a while, the amount of equipment we needed for Réyan but couldn't get from the NHS started to mount up.

Eventually, Harnish and I reasoned that this wasn't anyone else's money; no one else would receive it if we didn't take it. It's offered to us alone, and we really should take it. When we received the first payment, we immediately bought a shower chair and started getting a bit excited about the equipment we could buy for Réyan. There are so many amazing inventions. It became a real opportunity to give Réyan a better standard of life and the best life possible. We also save what we can of it for him so there's a nice little nest egg when he's older. I wish we'd claimed benefits from the start now, even though the benefits system is a bit of a maze and the forms alone seem specifically designed to confuse and take the maximum amount of time. Even if you're lucky enough to be quite well off, I say take what you're offered as soon as you're able, but try to use it as a bonus for extra special things or your child's future.

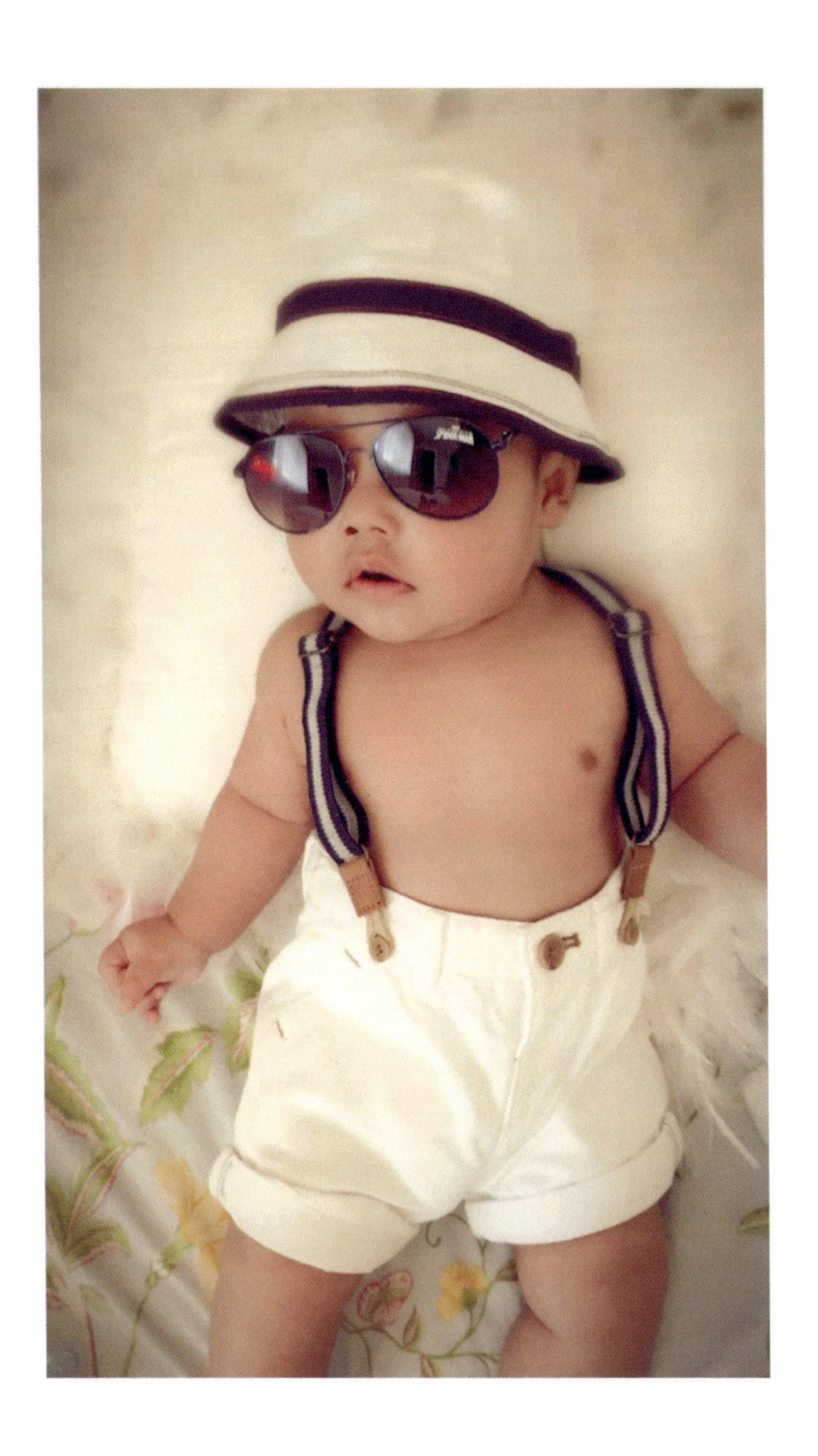

CHAPTER 4: RÉYAN'S DAY

Is there a gene for waking up full of beans? If so, Réyan and I share it. I never wake up on the wrong side of the bed, ever, nor does he. Réyan wakes up happy and full of smiles, and the morning starts with kisses and cuddles in bed while we do his exercises. Recently, he's also started telling us if he's tired and needs more sleep or if he's had a good sleep or he had a dream or whatever.

To get him up, we ask him to roll onto his side and swing his legs to the side of his bed, and we help him sit up. He doesn't have balance, but he gets up, and we hold him upright, and he looks around as we explain to him what his day is going to be about. We sign and ask if he wants to go to the toilet, and he says yes or no, and I ask if he has a wet nappy. I think it's very important to ask – I don't like just touching his nappy without his consent. He will check and say 'yes' or 'no' and nine out of ten times, he's right.

There's a second set of exercises in the lounge. Réyan picks which programme he wants to watch while we do tummy time and lots of speaking. Then, more choices – Réyan is in control of his life as much as possible. What breakfast would he like? Porridge, toast, banana on top? At the weekend, he can choose to go out for breakfast or have waffles. We've recently bought him a special spoon; the handle is diagonal, so he doesn't need to turn his wrist. It's been a game-changer.

Next, we try to get him to stand up in the bathroom. We've refused a hoist so far because I know we'll come to rely on it. When it gets too tough and we've tried every single thing, that's when we'll get a hoist, but right now, even though it's hard work to pick up a five-year-old, we're managing. I get him to stand by his bed holding a rail, and we say, 'Oops, you're going to fall' or 'Oh no, Mama's going to hurt her back,' and he'll try all the harder. And then I say, 'Wow! You're so tall! Aren't you tall!' – in that time, I've quickly put a nappy on.

A quick diversion here: can you imagine trying to do this in a public washroom or toilet cubicle? And not just when your child is five, but when he's eight or ten. There are no facilities for children like Réyan – not even in disabled lavatories or changing rooms aimed at able-bodied babies. This is where I find myself sobbing behind Réyan's wheelchair so he doesn't see me upset. Or when someone who has parked in a disabled parking and we have needed it the most. i am aware how some disabilities are not physical but still. They've been completely overlooked. I've written to my local council to ask them to consider the problems we have and what can be done to help.

Back to our morning routine, and after the nappy change, I get Réyan to lie on the floor and use his hand to pull his trousers up. I noticed M&S and Sainsburys introduced these lovely shirts with Velcro around their wrists, and it's brilliant for any child who has problems with fine motor skills. They stocked them last year but then stopped, so my mum's actually taken all his shirts, removed the buttons and put Velcro on them so he's able to help dress himself. Then he's very proud of himself, and he wants to have a look in the mirror. Mirror work is very important because Réyan needs to see himself and understand what his body is doing and correct himself or even try to.

The way people often work out that special needs children, including Réyan, have a condition is the way they open their mouths and move their heads from side to side. It just looks different. So I say to Réyan, 'Can you see if you can close your mouth? You don't see Mama sitting with her mouth open, look around and try your hardest. I believe in you. But that's between him and me – I wouldn't say that in public or with anyone else present. But if I can manage to just bring him closer to the world other children inhabit, then I will because it will make life better for Réyan.

I was initially told there would be deformities to Réyan's face, and I remembered some of my patients on the stroke ward and looked up pictures of children on the internet. I thought, 'Oh my goodness, I can manage it, but can it be managed in the real world?' As I said before, I wouldn't change Réyan for the world – but I would change the world for Réyan, and if I can't do that, we just carry on doing the best we can.

So, I say, 'You've got your mouth really wide open, can you feel that? I'll show you in the mirror.' And I open my mouth wide, and I say, 'When Mama sits, do I sit like this?' This is all done in a very soft way. 'Do you think you can do the same as me?'

These days, if Réyan has his mouth open, without a word from anyone, he will slowly, slowly, close it. It makes me smile, but I also want to hug him, cry and kiss him all at once because

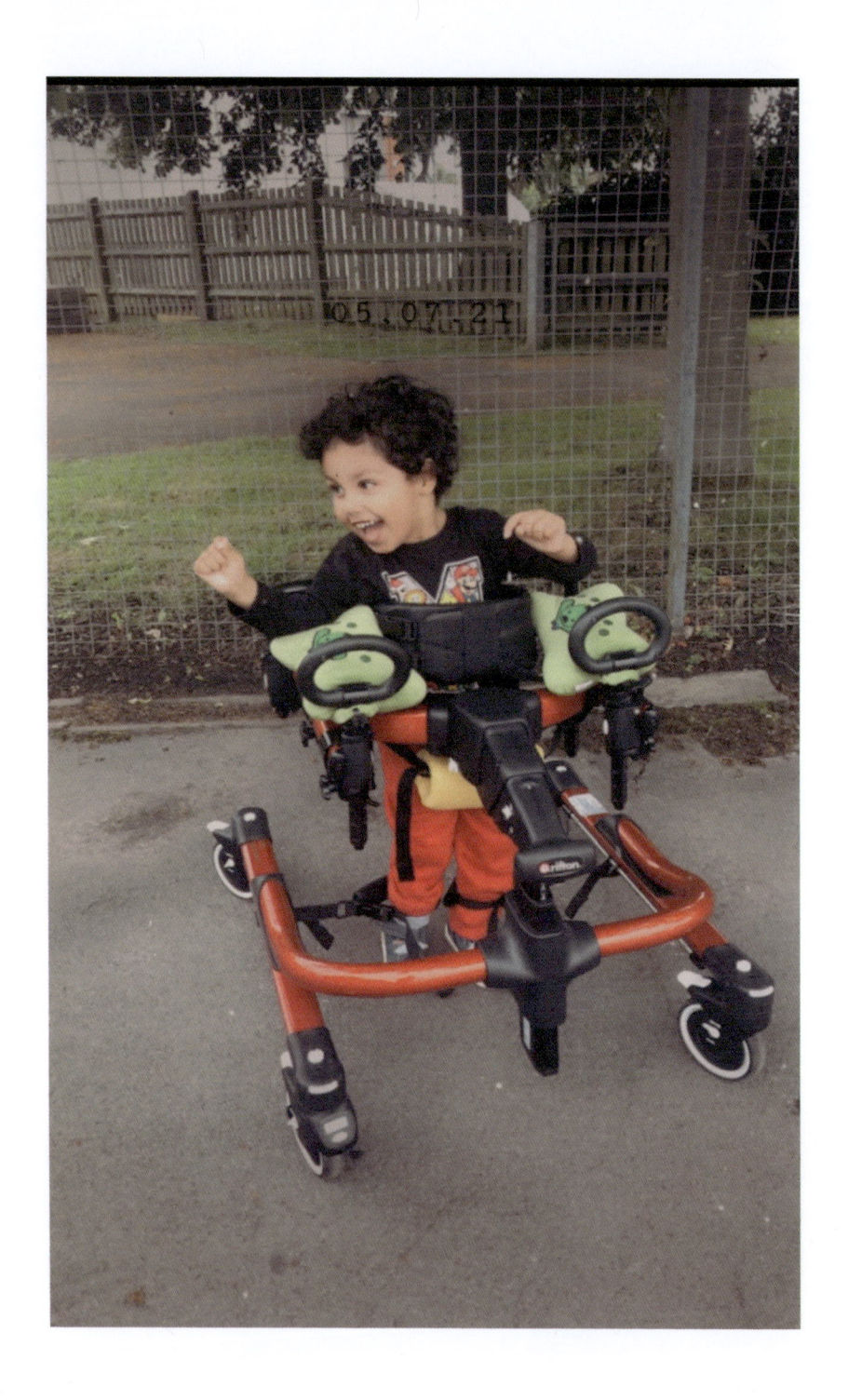

he's such a trier. He's such a wonderful boy. He teaches me so much.

Sometimes when I'm dressing him, Harnish may say just let him be; let him choose a bib that doesn't go with his clothes or let his hair stand on end or whatever. But I feel he already looks a bit muddled, and if we can avoid him looking any more so – if his hair is tidy and he has the right bib – then although he'll always stand out because of his needs, people's reactions will also be less visible, and again, that's nicer for Réyan. It's a case of making him as acceptable as possible to the world so that the world can welcome him. We have enough mountains to climb – let's try to smooth the path when we can.

What's more, I want him to take pride in how he looks so he can look in the mirror and like what he sees there. It's all part of developing that sense of self; knowing who they are and what they like is something that all children need. I'm still me if I rush out of the door with a frayed top and unbrushed hair. But I'm a slightly better me if I put on something clean and ironed and my hair is neat – that's all I'm trying to do for Réyan.

Now we're ready for the day, which usually means school. We have a special needs car through the Motability scheme, which means we can fit all our equipment. But Réyan uses a regular car seat. The special needs ones sell for between £10,00–£13,000, but this regular one cost us £100 from Amazon, and it's great. It has lots of support, which we bolster even more with rolled towels, etc., and, crucially, it swings around so we can get at him easily. Thank goodness too for the 'GoTo Chair'. I can honestly say this bit of kit has been life-changing. It travels with us everywhere. The GoTo Chair enables Réyan to go on a swing, sit with us on the floor, go to a posh restaurant, leave the wheelchair at the door and sit on a normal chair.

After school, Réyan's choice is always to go to a restaurant to eat – but obviously, we can't do that too often. When we get home, we change his clothes, wash his hands and face and, by that time, he's often very tired and just wants to relax and daydream a bit. However, we do encourage him to show us what he did at school, which he does through pointing at picture cards or signing. Sometimes neither of us knows how to sign a word, so we go on YouTube, play the video and learn how to sign it together. Réyan takes me to YouTube, and he knows fully how to use the iPad and I type in '**Makaton how to**'. It's brilliant, and there are hundreds of videos.

Réyan also gets half an hour on the iPad to do anything he wants. We always get takeaway on Friday nights, and we've shown him how it works and how to do it. One time he was very quiet and busy and then started to point at the door, and I said, 'You're right, it's nearly time for Daddy to come home.' But he said, 'No' and was pointing to the iPad. I was a bit confused but didn't think too much of it. Suddenly the doorbell goes, and Réyan is so excited, giggling away and smiling from ear to ear. It's Deliveroo with pizzas. Five pizzas! When Harnish did come back, he said, 'Someone's hungry!' Yes dear, not me. Your son. And Réyan was signing eating and chuckling. I think we can file that under the heading 'Victims of Our Own Success'!

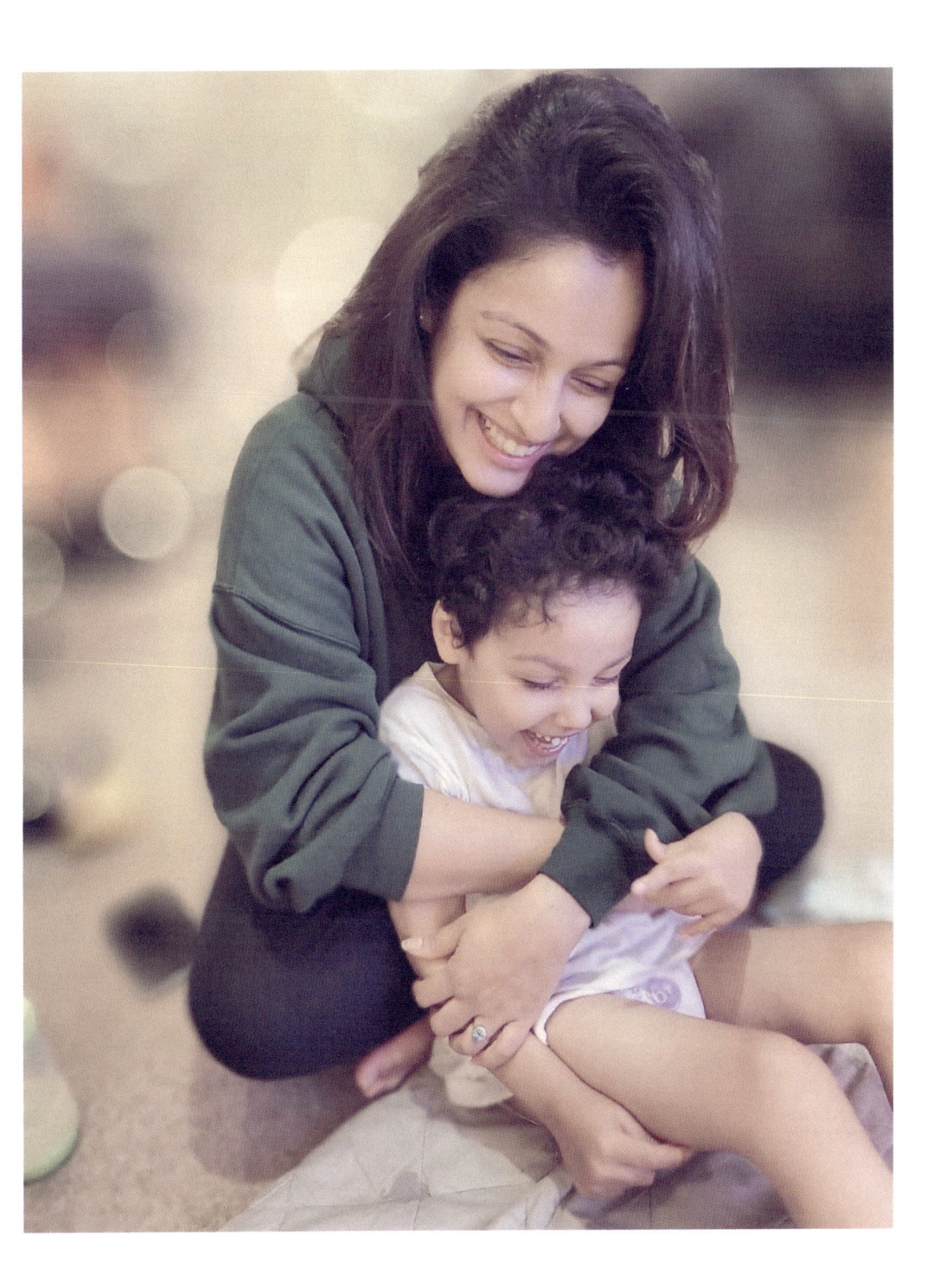

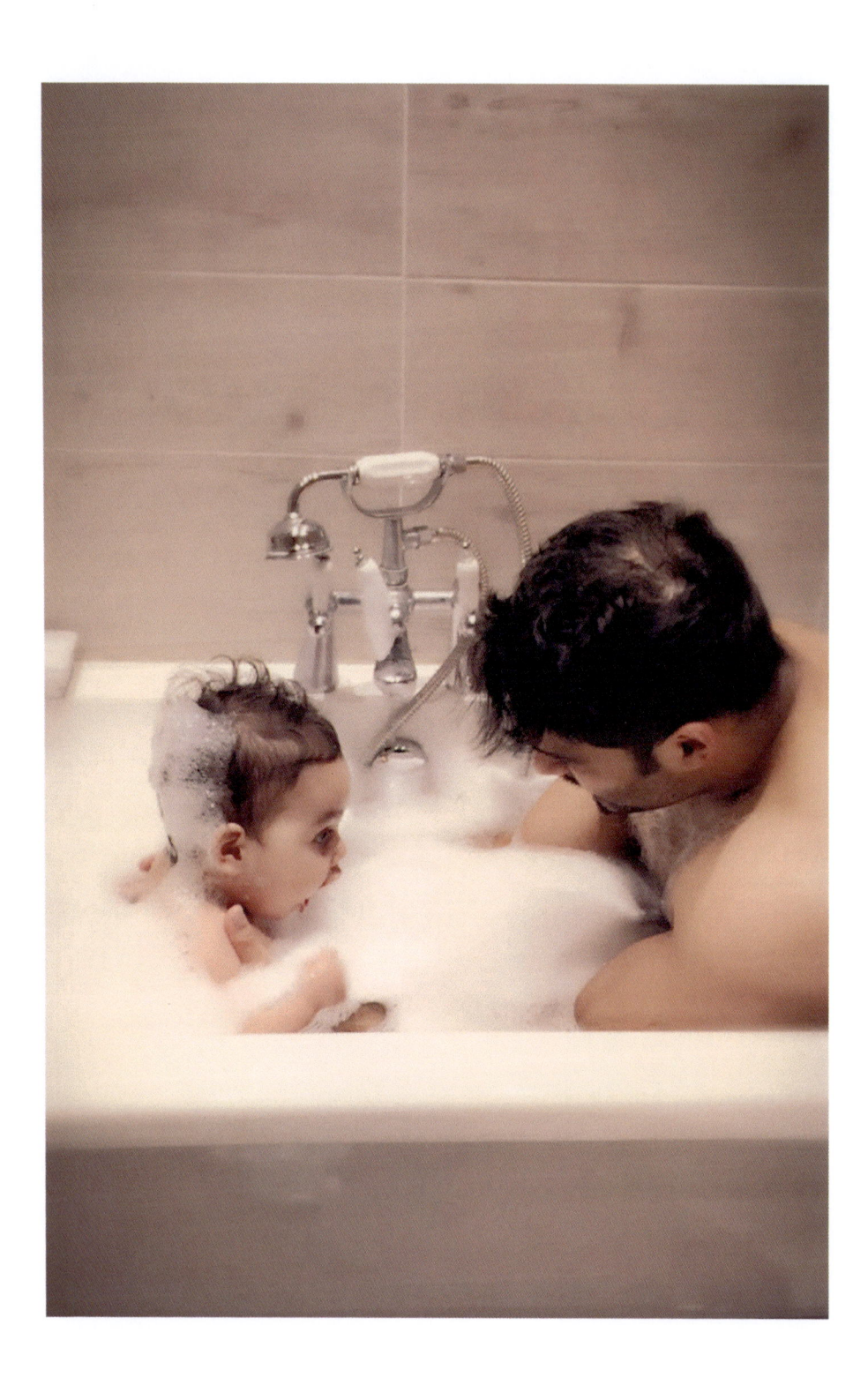

Réyan does play with toys, but so many are just totally unsuitable for differently-abled children. There can be nothing worse than being given a bright new toy and not being able to use it. I was wondering what I was going to do, a course in engineering perhaps? Then I discovered Re-map. They are a wonderful group of ex-servicemen who modify toys for children like Réyan. They sit in a room wearing bow ties and working on the toys like a group of full-sized elves!

Thursday is pamper time: I set up a bowl of hot bubbly water, Réyan gets a drink of his choice and I give him a manicure and pedicure and put oil in his hair. I call him 'Sir Réyan' and say, 'Would you like this or that?' and he's just so excited. It's lovely times like these, even if they're only half an hour, that makes everything worthwhile.

We then move towards evening, and I ask Réyan what he fancies for dinner, and he'll help me with the cooking. We wait for Daddy, and candles and music are always on the cards for dinner. Nowadays, if we go to someone's for dinner, Réyan always looks around for the candles and music. I played him a lot of jazz when I was pregnant, and even now, he still likes to listen to it. He's very sensitive to music; it stops him crying if he's upset, his muscles relax and his spasticity eases when he listens to soft, calming music.

Bath time is Daddy time, and it's always lots of fun. When Réyan was very small and couldn't sit up in the bath because of his condition, I remember one time Harnish said, 'I'm fed up with these stupid chairs that don't work for him. He's not enjoying it, nor are we. What can we do?' Then the pair of us thought, 'sod it,' and we both got in the bath with him! And that's how we did it; one held him, one played. We ended up getting this massive bath, way too big for our bathroom, then a bubble machine and a disco light – we just went for it!

Now it's exclusively Harnish's time. I can't physically hold Réyan anymore, and I was always nervous, but they have a ball. Réyan does have a harness and a special chair these days, but Harnish makes it so much fun he forgets he's in a chair. Among other things, Réyan uses his finger to pop the bubbles – another sensory and physical activity. He has to really concentrate to use his hand accurately and loves the sense of achievement when he's popped a bubble. I always, always, ask myself, 'How can I teach him something here but in a fun way so that he'll not realise he's learning?'

So, that's the nuts and bolts of our routine. Days out, let alone holidays, require an altogether different level of planning. We'll sometimes see somewhere online and think it looks amazing, but then we start with, 'How do we get him there?', 'What if there are no slopes?' and 'OK, what if I carry Réyan and you carry the wheelchair?' – and there are fewer opportunities for even that arrangement as Réyan gets bigger. Sometimes we'll call the place and ask if they can help; they are often very nice but just haven't got the staff available to open gates or whatever for us. So, after getting all excited, the trip just fizzles out.

Then there's the perennial problem of people who aren't disabled using the disabled parking bays. That really hurts. I actually feel it as physical pain. I've had to leave a shopping centre before because there's been no disabled parking, or I've maybe waited for half an hour – kept Réyan busy in the car, brought him into the front with me to do things with him – then we see someone come out to their car in the disabled space, and there's no disability and no badge either (as I recognise some disabilities are hidden). Or else we make it into the centre and the lift's broken. It just really, really, gets to me. We've packed up and planned, and Réyan's excited, and then we have to go all the way home without doing anything.

It's great that so many outdoor playgrounds now have equipment for children with special needs, but again, sometimes we've had the whole palaver of getting the wheelchair through the park, only to find there are 10 normal swings and one special needs swing, and there's a huge crowd of kids on the special needs swing. I say to Réyan, 'Let them have a go. It's because your swing is extra fun; that's why everyone wants a go.' So we wait, and sometimes we're just ignored. In one instance, we'd been waiting a particularly long time, and I asked a mother if she could persuade her fully-abled child to play on something else so we could just use it for 10 minutes, and she shouted at me. Réyan was starting to look anxious and worried, so we just left. People don't seem to understand we only have that one swing; they have the whole playground. We have now found a park with lots of equipment for special needs children, and it's brilliant, but it requires quite a lot of Googling to find places like that. You have to put in the research hours, and it's a needle in a haystack.

When we want to book a holiday, we know from the outset that insurance will be more expensive, and if we're flying, we need to go business as we just can't cope in economy – the narrower seats aren't suitable for Réyan. That's before we think about meds, food, Réyan's exercise regime or what equipment to take, and before we're even halfway down the list, we end up wondering if we should go in the first place. But we realise we're lucky to both be working, and it's a privilege to be able to afford these breaks. Many SEN parents never go on holiday.

It's a really tough world out there for us. I remember one time trudging through an airport, Harnish and I carrying Réyan, his wheelchair and his car seat all the way to the furthest gate. No sitting in the club lounge or browsing duty-free for us. We started to bicker, and I felt the room closing in. I'm not religious, but usually, I feel there is something out there. At that moment, I felt truly abandoned – there was no spiritual guidance, just an overwhelming emotion that this wasn't fair. But then, I thought of Réyan, because who has he got if not me. I pulled myself out of my dark place, and on we went.

I am Réyan's physiotherapist, his speech and language therapist, his potty-training therapist, his drooling therapist – you name it, that's me! It's a lonely place being an SEN parent. One piece of the jigsaw of our day that I haven't mentioned is the screaming and the crying. Never out loud, never in front of Réyan. I used to scream into my hands when I washed my face in the mornings. I cried and cried in the shower. How lonely is that when the only place you can cry is under the shower? It's been five years. I'm managing – my toolbox is serving me well; I have everything I need, but I'm really bunged up sometimes, with a lump in my throat that's so big it's difficult to breathe.

But then I'll be talking to Réyan, and I'll say, 'Where's your heart?' and he points to mine and then to his. We've not taught him to do that. That's him – he's done that. And that's the final bit of what makes up Réyan's day and mine: I'm in buckets. I'm in buckets every day because of this boy who's so beautiful inside and out.

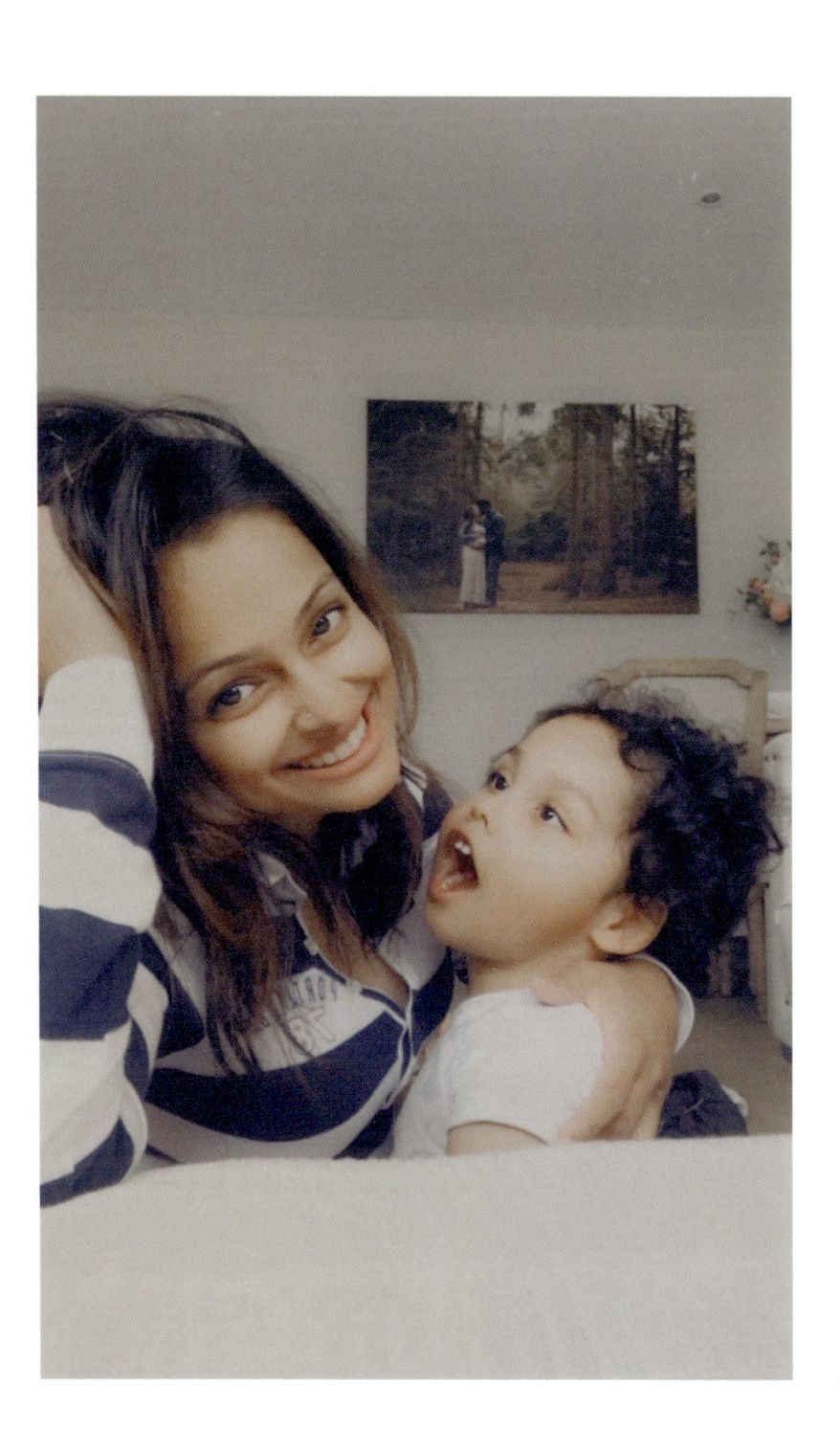

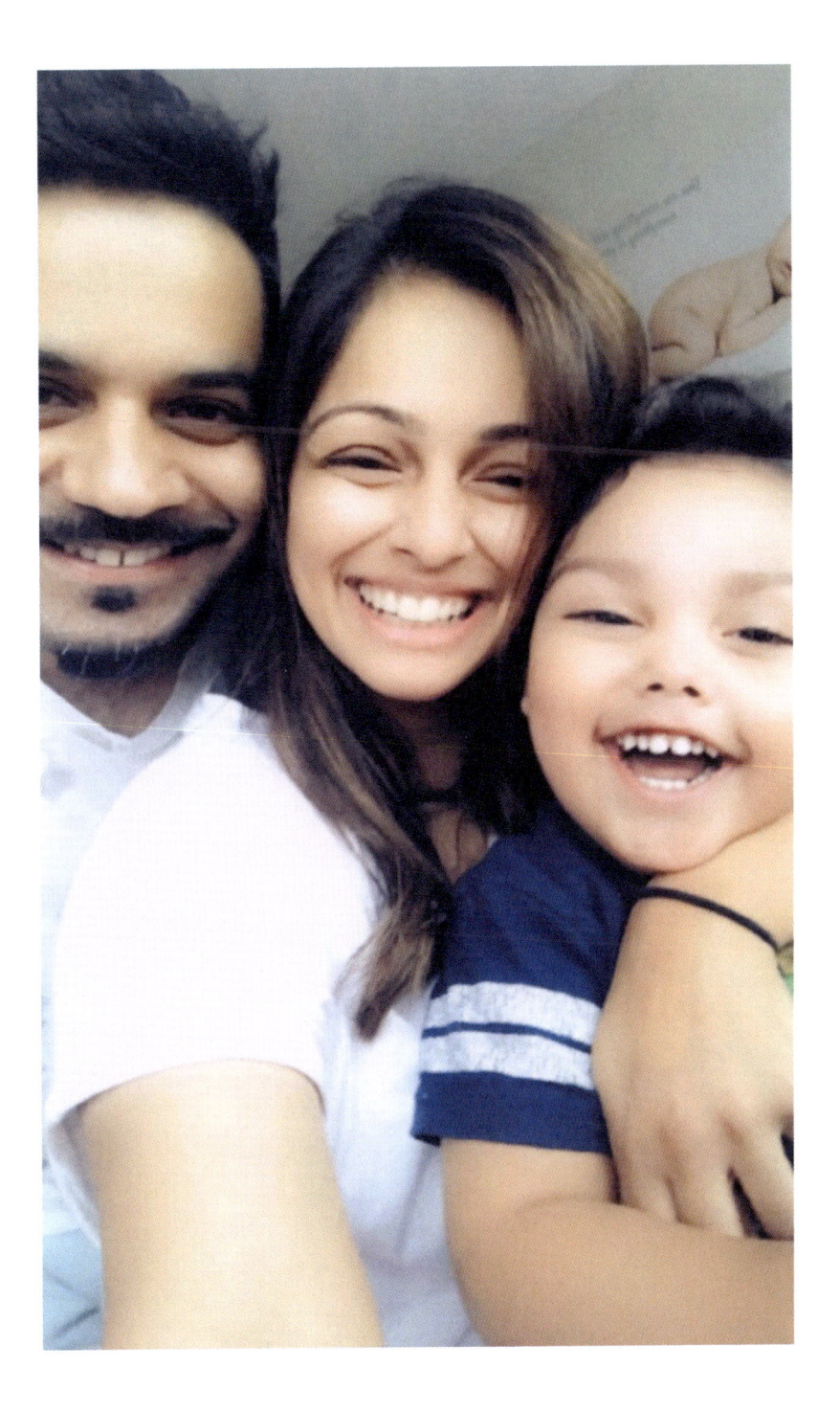

CHAPTER 5: THE 50-THOUSAND-POUND GAMBLE

In the autumn of 2019, Réyan, Harnish and I, along with my wonderful, unbelievably supportive parents, abandoned our lives for three months so Réyan could undergo stem cell treatment in India. The cells would be injected through the spine as a lumber puncture process to regenerate the cells.

It was a 50-thousand-pound gamble. My parents had been extremely generous and given us some money for the operation. Harnish and I also used up all our savings, and the final portion came from 18 months of fundraising. Cake sales, runs, out in the cold selling hot drinks – you name it, we did it – raising a total of £17,000 towards the treatment. We're so grateful to everyone who supported us.

Two years later, we still don't know if it's worked. We'll probably never know, and that's fine. I had hopes but no expectations. I just felt in my gut as a mother that if there was any chance of it working, we needed to try. Even if the stem cells only improved Réyan's life by five or 10 per cent, that's still better than doing nothing. And if we'd not done it, I think I would always have wondered if things could have been better for us.

It wasn't a leap in the dark, though. I did a lot of research, as did my parents, and I am lucky to have a number of friends who are doctors who also did a bit of digging. One even went to look at the institute in India and check it out for us. I, too, went

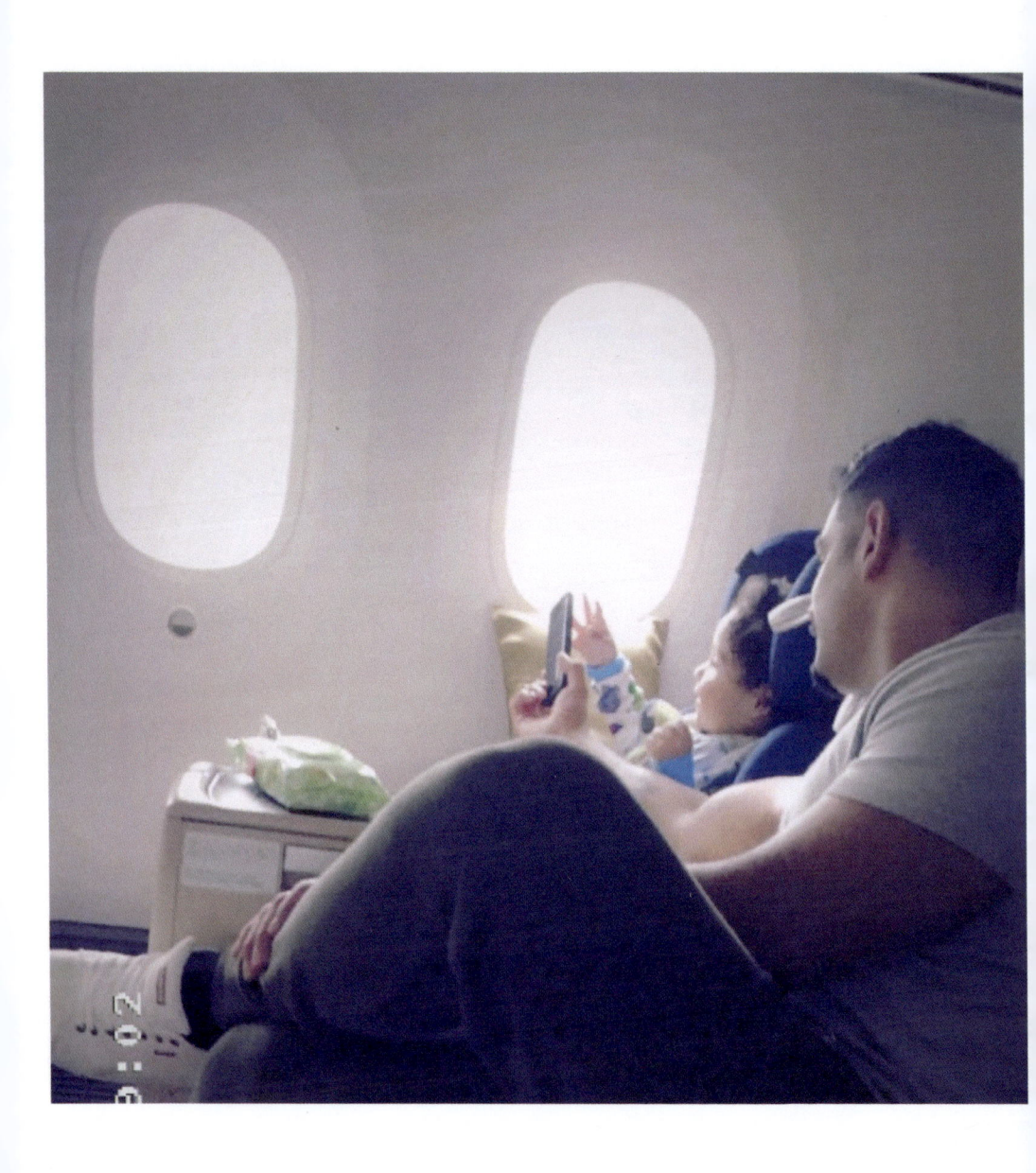

out six months beforehand to look at it and watch how they harvest the cells. I wanted to be sure it was the right place before we committed to the treatment. We chose India because our research showed that, while American clinics seem to have the most success with children who have blood cancers or tumours, India led the field for treating cerebral palsy.

I also spoke to a number of NHS doctors. A very close friend of mine from day 1. Every one in my family adores him and I cherish our friendship. They have to be very careful what they say, but from my medical background, I could decipher what they were trying to tell me. The bottom line was there was no disadvantage to the treatment. There might not be any actual advantage, but the cells couldn't cause any harm in themselves. I work with some lovely professionals who ran through the pros and cons with me – both as a doctor and as a dad.

Our network of friends and colleagues really was invaluable. The treatment works by taking some stem cells and injecting them into his brain, like a lumbar puncture procedure. The idea is that they seed and grow and help to repair some of the damage. It's risky only in that all general anaesthetics are risky, and Réyan had already had one of those and been fine with no adverse or allergic reactions. Once I realised that there were no disadvantages to the treatment, I was determined to go for it.

That's not to say I didn't have moments of doubt. My faith as a mother was very strong, but I did find myself repeating (even though I wasn't sure who I was talking to), 'If it doesn't work out, then so be it, but don't leave us in a worse state . . . Please,

please, don't do that.' In my head, the words *what if, what if . . . what if he ends up worse . . .* went round and round. But I knew that if we did nothing, then it was guaranteed the 'what ifs' would last a lifetime.

One of the advantages of choosing India was that the cost of living there is much cheaper than here (or indeed if we'd gone to America). We could afford physio every day, which was amazing. In Britain, an hour of private physio costs £90, but in India, it was £10 for two hours a day – there's just no comparison!

There was also no comparison between the Réyan that left for India and the child we have now. He was a changed boy when he came home, and today he achieves so much more than we were told would ever be possible. But is it the stem cells? I can't answer that.

All I do know is how that brain scan looked for the areas concerned with motor skills and particularly, communication. I can see those grey, black and white areas, but I also know what Réyan can actually do. I was most concerned about communication – if there's no communication, that's really tough. But what the original doctors meant by communication was speaking, and although I accept we're a long way from that, Réyan has fantastic eye contact, he can use an iPad, he can sign – he's communicating all the time.

But perhaps those two months with physio every day, our continuing private physio, the swimming, the stretching routine – plus all the effort Harnish and I put in – have had just as much effect. Harnish would be the first to admit he found it difficult to really give Réyan his all in the early days. He says he felt like he wanted to do better but didn't know how. It was hard to express himself, but he felt parenting just wasn't coming naturally. Then all of a sudden – later than me – he connected. Let's face it, we're all learning each day, and Réyan didn't come with a manual. As parents, we sometimes don't know what we're doing, but as long as we do it from the heart, the child can only benefit.

It wasn't long after we returned from India that the first of the coronavirus lockdowns were imposed, so Harnish spent even more time with Réyan, and it made their bond even stronger. We saw a difference with Réyan and really noticed Harnish's input. Harnish says he thinks lots of dads – whether their children are differently-abled or not – don't understand how much impact they can have.

So maybe the improvements we see in Réyan are a combination of everything that has just gelled and worked together: the stem cells, the physio, us and, of course, him – Réyan himself. By God, this boy loves to try!

For instance, if he wants to pick something up, but he can't quite manage it, he'll try again and again. He's so determined. His face goes funny, his other hand will have spasticity and he's drooling, drooling, drooling, but still, he keeps trying, and he's so tired by the time he gets there. But then I'll be clapping and whooping because I'm so pleased he's done it, and he's smiling and saying, 'Oooh, oooh, oooh!' like 'You were watching me?!' and he's so pleased, and I say, 'Well done, you can do it! You really can do it!' and he's all 'Yeah, yeah . . .'

The human brain is amazing. It's so **plastic**, and everything can be tweaked. We'll probably never understand the full story, but I do want to know what's going on in that brain of Réyan's. I'm so curious to know and learn more about him. I ask him all the time, what's going on in that beautiful mind of yours. Tell me. Show me. Let's explore together. Teach me to see through your eyes and your mind.

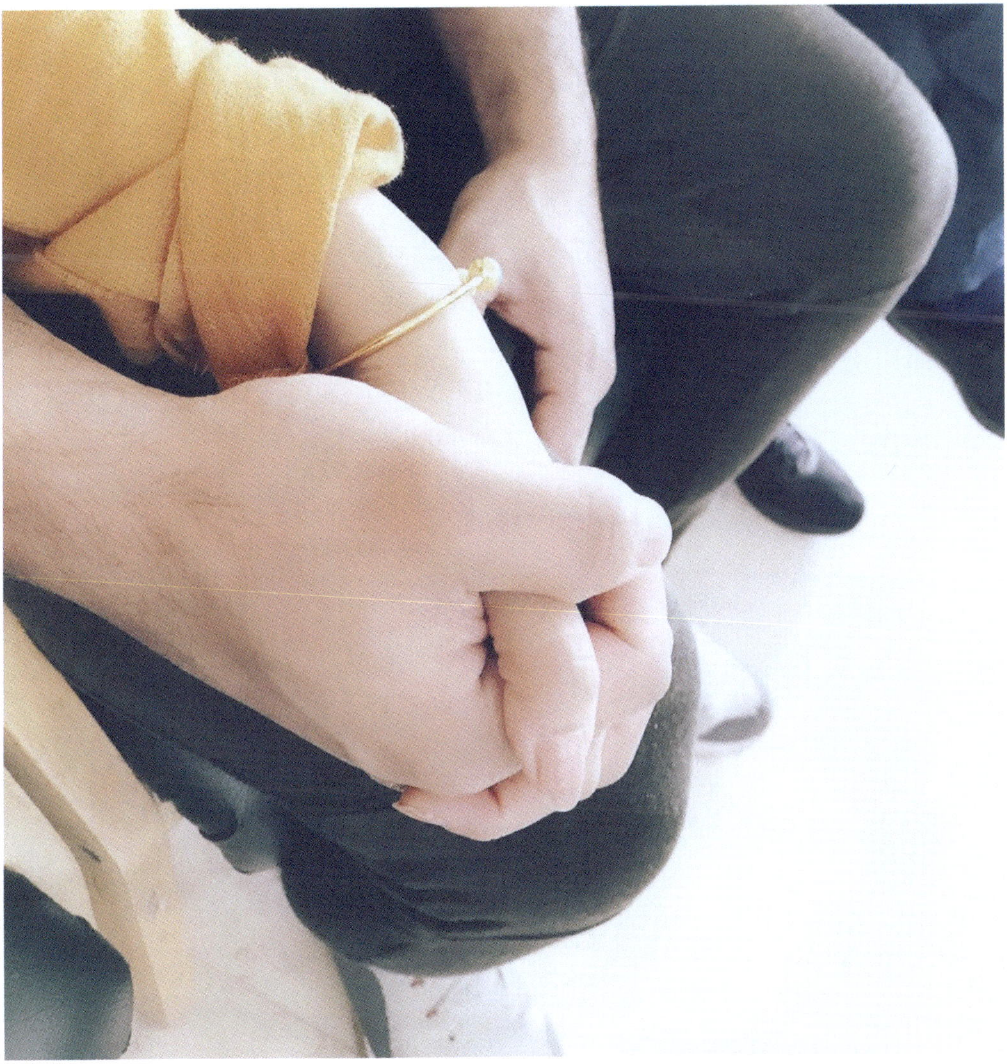

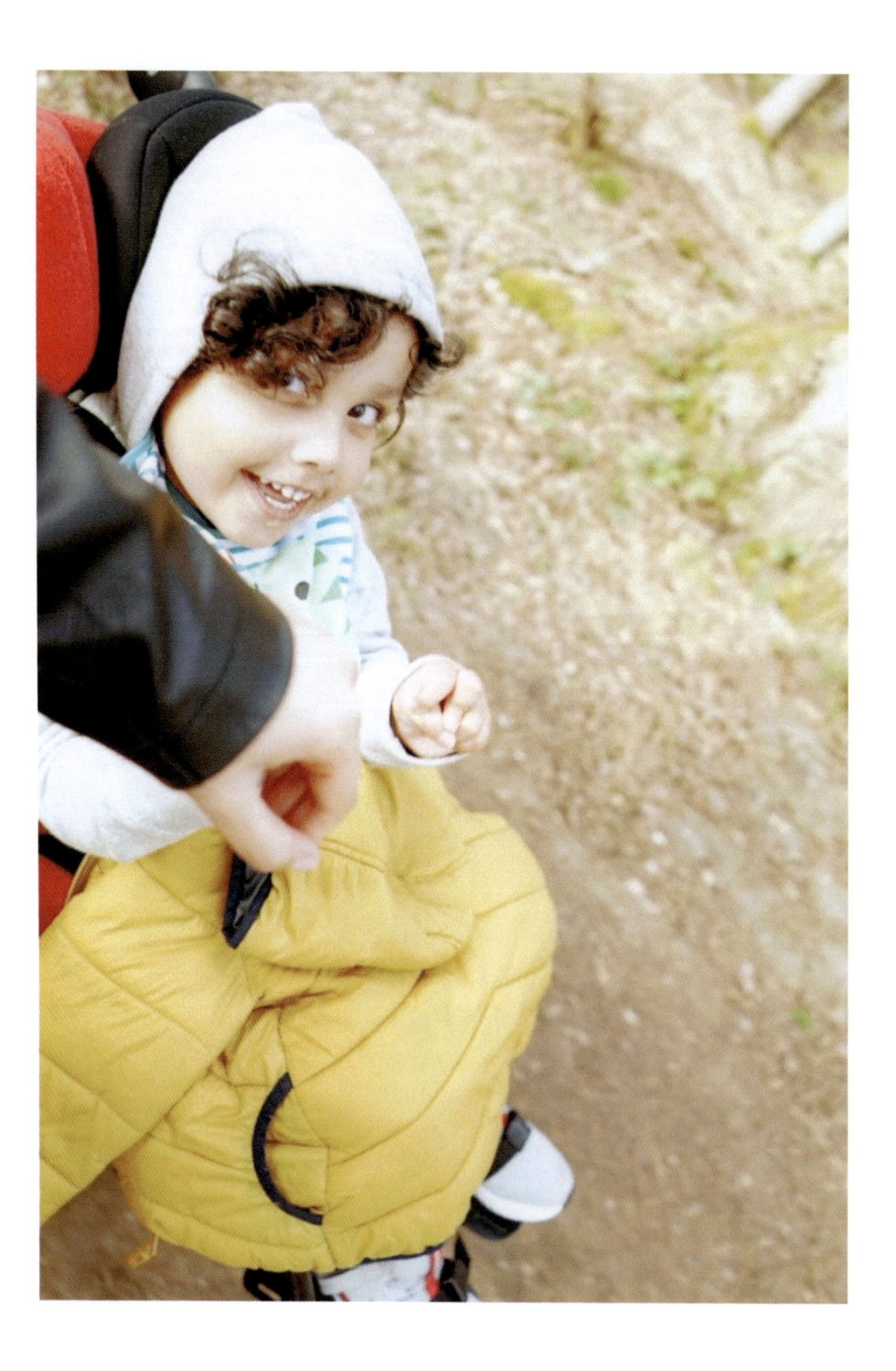

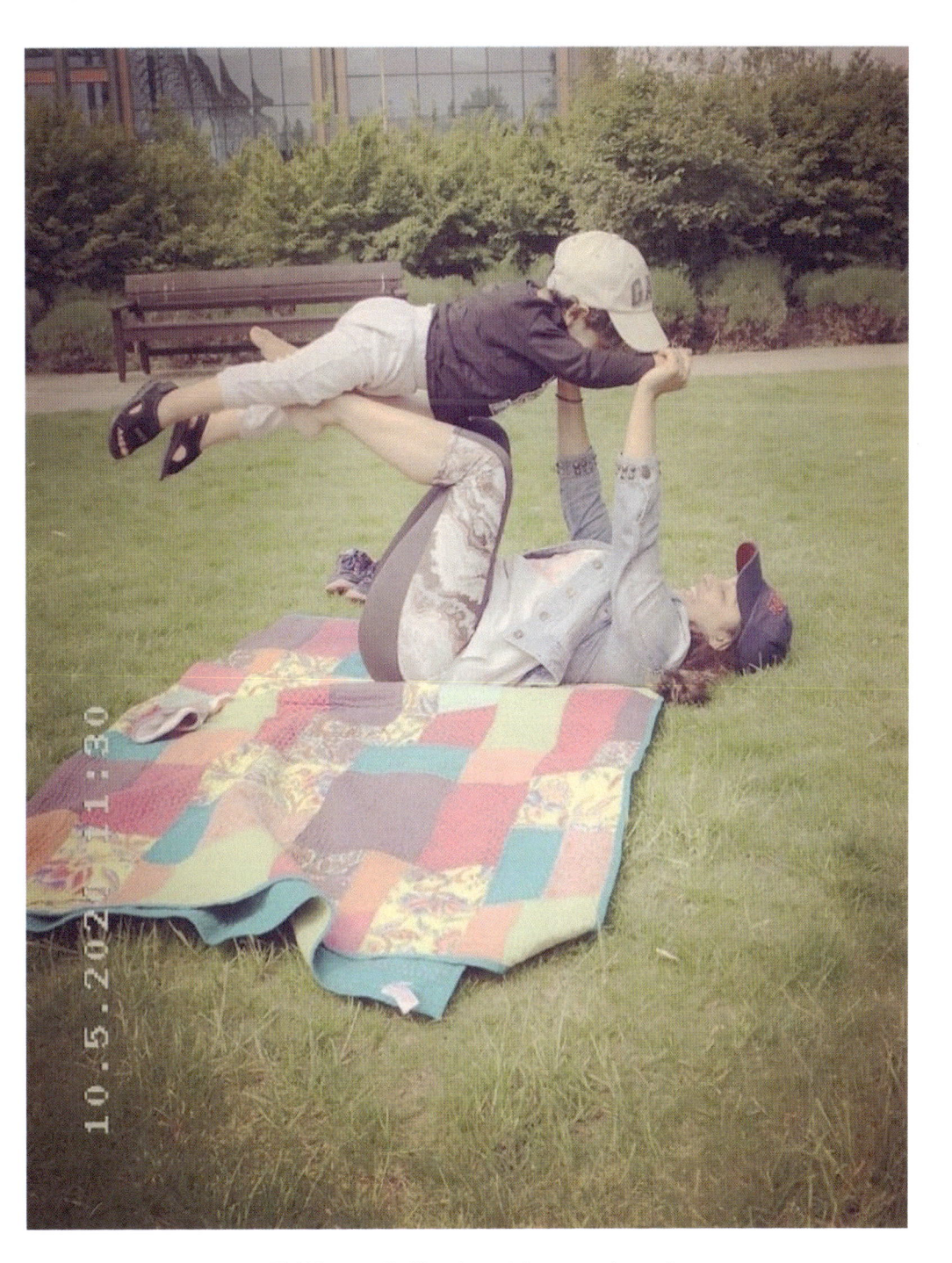

Fly high my son I will continue to help you spread your wings

CHAPTER 6: SUNFLOWER BOY

Now seems a good time to introduce the final member of our family: Oliver. Anyone who knows Reyan well knows Oliver. Here's how he came into our life. Réyan's right hand works much better than his left, so naturally, he favours that one. He's got pretty good grip, so he uses that hand and his one very good finger for the most intricate things. Sometimes he will let go of things when he doesn't mean to or when his concentration slips, so I ordered him an 'Easy Grip' strap to help him hold a pen. It's a little strap that goes round him, and then you put the pen in. We've started doing some dot-to-dots together.

As I've mentioned, Réyan learns differently than fully-functioning children, so teaching him in the normal way is like a brainstorm for him. Sometimes we need to turn the volume down and just do something very slowly and quietly – and do it together rather than him being formally taught.

It's important that Réyan still moves and tries to use his left hand, or its spasticity will increase, and the difference in functionality between the two hands will widen. But all my usual methods were hitting a brick wall, and in trying and trying to get Réyan to use that left hand, we overwhelmed him. He was constantly being reminded, 'Use your left hand' and he got totally fed up. It got to the point where Réyan was sticking his tongue out at his left hand and would hide it under the table. He was just very embarrassed of that hand, and it was lowering his confidence in general.

Then I remembered one of my stroke patients who'd had a bad bleed on the right-hand side of his brain, affecting the left side of his body. So, in hospital, his table was on his right side, and everyone always approached him to talk on the right side. However, once or twice a day, I began sitting on his left side to write up his notes or have a little chat. He couldn't really turn that way at all, but every day it was a little bit easier for him, and after six months, he could turn to that side. I also started occasionally moving a table with one or two light things on it to the left side to encourage him to reach out, and he did eventually start using that hand a little bit. But it's slow progress and requires huge amounts of patience and perseverance – there's no quick fix. I remember arguing the case in team meetings and saying, 'Yes, the right side is going to be the most functional side, and we definitely need to concentrate on that, but let's not give up altogether on the left.'

It's the same with Réyan. We know the right hand is always going to be his functional one. But he was becoming almost scared of his other hand and kind of disowning it, and that was no good long term. So, I decided to call it Oliver. I said to Réyan, 'Guess what?' – whenever I say that, he knows it's something exciting, so he's really listening.

'Guess what, you've got a new friend. And he's called Oliver! You know your hand? Well, I've found out he's called Oliver! And we've been calling it "leftie" all this time! No wonder he wasn't moving – we've been calling him the wrong name!'

Réyan totally bought into the story of 'Oliver', so now we say, 'Oh, you can't just keep using one hand, Oliver is going to feel left out' or 'Perhaps we should include Oliver in this' or 'Let's not just use one hand, it's not fair on Oliver,' and he tries really, really hard to get that left hand working. Sometimes I would discreetly move his arm for him, so he doesn't realise it's me and thinks he's doing it – and that boost in confidence makes him try even harder. These days, he can hold food in his left hand, he's opening that hand up and he doesn't have to look at Oliver now – up he goes if he wants to raise that arm.

Réyan showed an interest in music from very early on, and a while ago, he started humming, but he kept getting shy and stopping when he realised we'd noticed. So I would sing at the top of my voice and then sign, 'Your turn,' and he would make noises, and I would exclaim, 'You didn't tell me you had such a voice!' and he would giggle and laugh, knowing I'm being over the top but also delighted with the praise. This Christmas, my mum and dad bought him a child's karaoke microphone with its own stand. Réyan loves it! We say, 'Oliver would love to help and be part of the band,' and Réyan opens his left hand and holds with two hands. So we have a house band, Réyan and his mate Oliver, and it's just the best, absolutely joyful.

So that's the story of Oliver and how we got Réyan moving his left hand. It's always going to be the helping arm, but it's so much more functional than it ever was. The whole Oliver project was also an exercise in teaching Réyan about looking after something, responsibility, interaction, love – he was learning so much as he worked to get that left arm moving.

It's very important Réyan doesn't lose track of his good hand, and we also make sure we celebrate his achievements with his right hand. In fact, any excuse for a party – one of the things my family certainly is good at is celebrating. When Réyan took his first steps, they decorated our house with balloons, and we had a family gathering to celebrate.

My parents have also helped Réyan become advanced for his years in one respect: he's already driving in his own car! They bought him a sit-in toy Mercedes that's the same as their car. At first, I was horrified they'd spent all this money on something he couldn't really use, but they said he could use the remote control and watch it go round, and he did enjoy that – he was able to control something! Then when we got the GoTo Chair, I was just praying it would fit – and it did! He can sit in and drive this car! The first time Réyan was going round in circles and just enjoying himself so much. When he gets really happy, his spasticity increases, so his jaw was just open; he couldn't close it! It's a wonderful feeling of independence for him. Mum and I had tears in our eyes watching him.

The challenges thrown up by the world sometimes make life with Réyan ultra-tough, but then, when everything clicks as it did that day, it's ultra-rewarding too. He really is a special boy in all senses of the word, and there seems to be a 'Réyan effect' that ripples out and touches all kinds of people.

The other day we were in Waitrose, and he was in his walker and also wanted to hold the basket, and he was choosing veg and other food to put in it. It isn't unusual for our 10-minute trip to turn into an hour, but he really enjoys it, and it's lots of

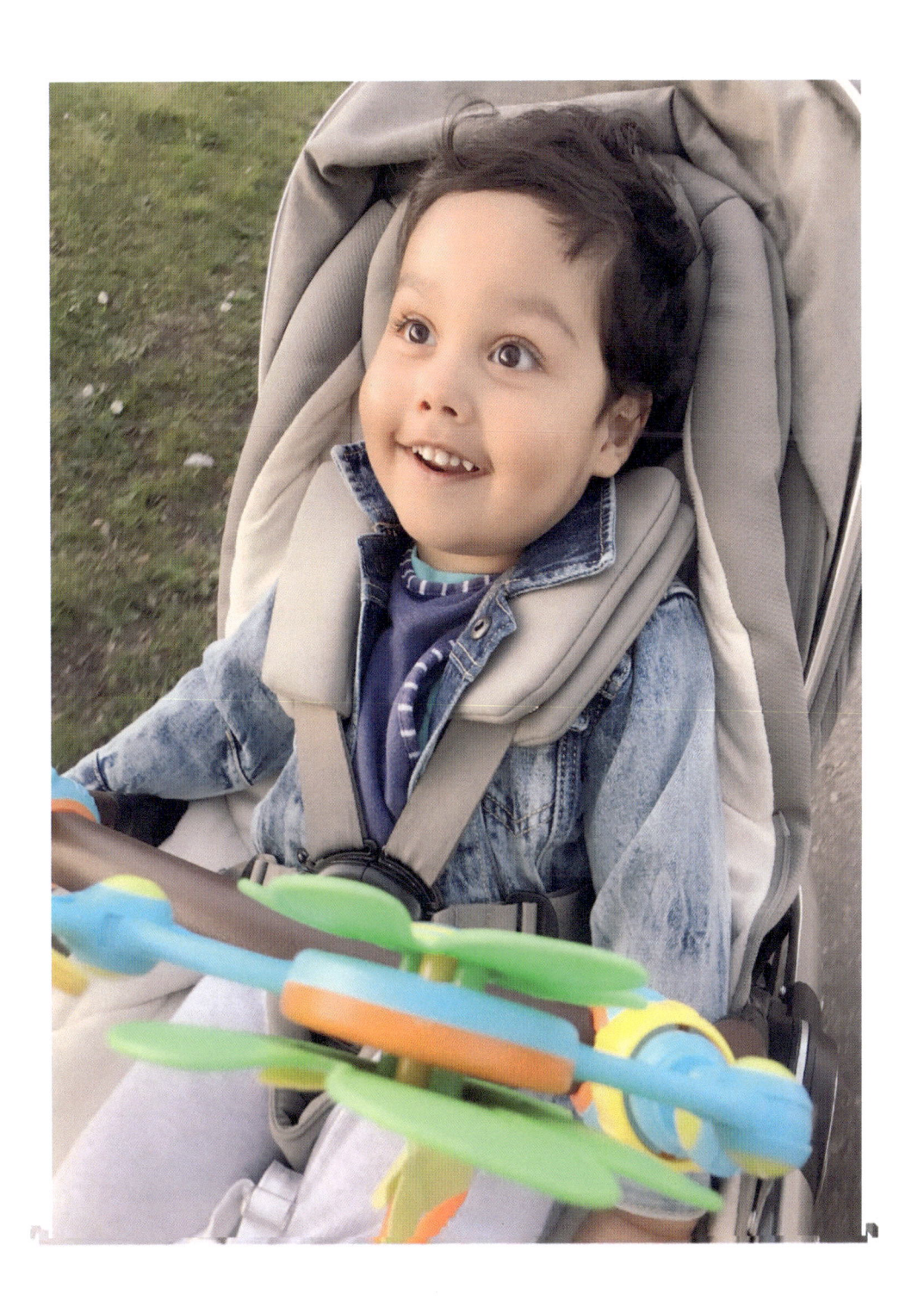

exercise. Réyan often wants to buy me flowers, and he was examining the display carefully when another shopper struck up a conversation. She asked to shake Réyan's hand and chatted to him, and he was nodding his head when she was asking about his day. As she straightened up she said to me, 'That's made my day. I was having a bad day, actually. There's so much wrong with the world, and everyone's always in a rush. But then I saw your boy walking around the shop, so happy and taking such care to pick nice flowers for you. He's incredible.'

I said I hope you'll have a better rest of the day, and we both walked on. Then at the tills, I saw her again, and she had a bunch of flowers in her hand, which she gave to Réyan, and he took them and signed thank you. She said, 'I've loved meeting you.'

Another time, we were in our local M&S, and whenever we go there, Réyan gets a treat from the cafe. It takes us a long time to walk through store, and that day he'd walked all the way, but by the time we had arrived, it was closed. Réyan does understand but I felt so bad for him. You have to get down to eye level, hold his hand and say, 'Look at me now. I need to tell you something important; we can't do this today, but maybe we'll buy a hat or do something else fun, or we'll see somewhere on the way home that you fancy popping into for a snack.'

So Harnish and I were down talking to him, and this lady who'd been sitting to one side came over and said she worked at the cafe. 'Please, let me open up for you,' she said and offered to toast a cheese sandwich for us. 'You're lucky you're so cute,' she said to Réyan with a smile. He was so excited, making all sorts of noises and signing 'thank you' when he got the sandwich. As we were leaving, I went back over and thanked the lady again, and she said, 'It wasn't much; there's no need for thanks.' And I said yes there was because we were heard without having to shout, and it was so lovely.

I do feel these days we've turned a corner and are making progress. I've started to think ahead to Réyan's future. Réyan said he wants to be a binman. I asked him why, and it's because he likes the sound of the truck – he hears them at the traffic lights long before we do – and also because they help clean the environment.

But he loves *Operation Ouch* on CBBC and loves our friends who are doctors who come to see us. They bought him a stethoscope, and I always say to him, 'Do you want to be a doctor?' and he says yes, then I ask him why, and he touches my heart and I say, 'You're going to make my heart better!' I've shown him how to take a temperature, and he's so interested. It's good for him to learn what people do and also for when he goes to the doctors to know what's happening. But any job he gets will be amazing – anything he can do. I look into the future in exactly the same way I would with a fully functioning child. There's no difference.

He is my sunflower boy. Just like sunflowers needing care and lots of sticks to help them grow. They do eventually turn into beautiful tall captivating living things. Just like Réyan.

REY'S OF SUNSHINE

Looking ahead just a year or two, I'd love to give Réyan a sibling. But we have some exciting plans ahead.

That's all to come.

For now I will continue to fight for Rèyan, continue being a crazy but happy Mumma, give him enough opportunities and choices daily. Continue to sing loud and make him laugh, continue to explore lovely restaurants, continue to drive on the side of lorries to give Rèyan some shade from the sun when we forget to put the sun screen up.

But I want to end where I started, with a message to Réyan:

My wonderful boy, my beautiful sunflower. I know life has been challenging so far, but one thing I am very certain about is loving you has been easy. I gave birth to you, but you have given me life. Nothing will stop me from giving you all I have because you are everything and everything is you.

Who knows how the future will pan out and what is down the line for our little family, but we have love, and we have patience, and that can conquer anything.

We got this.

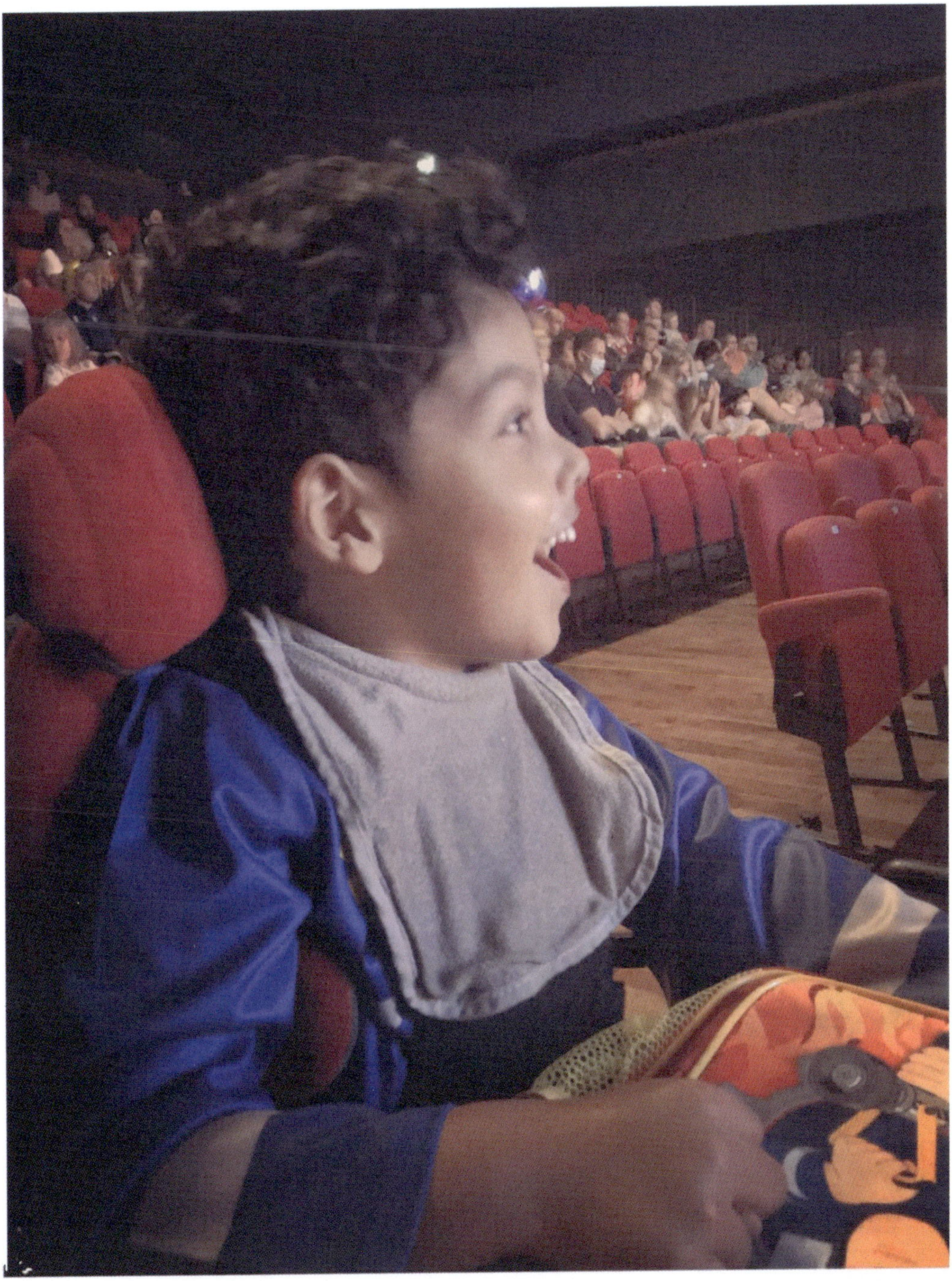

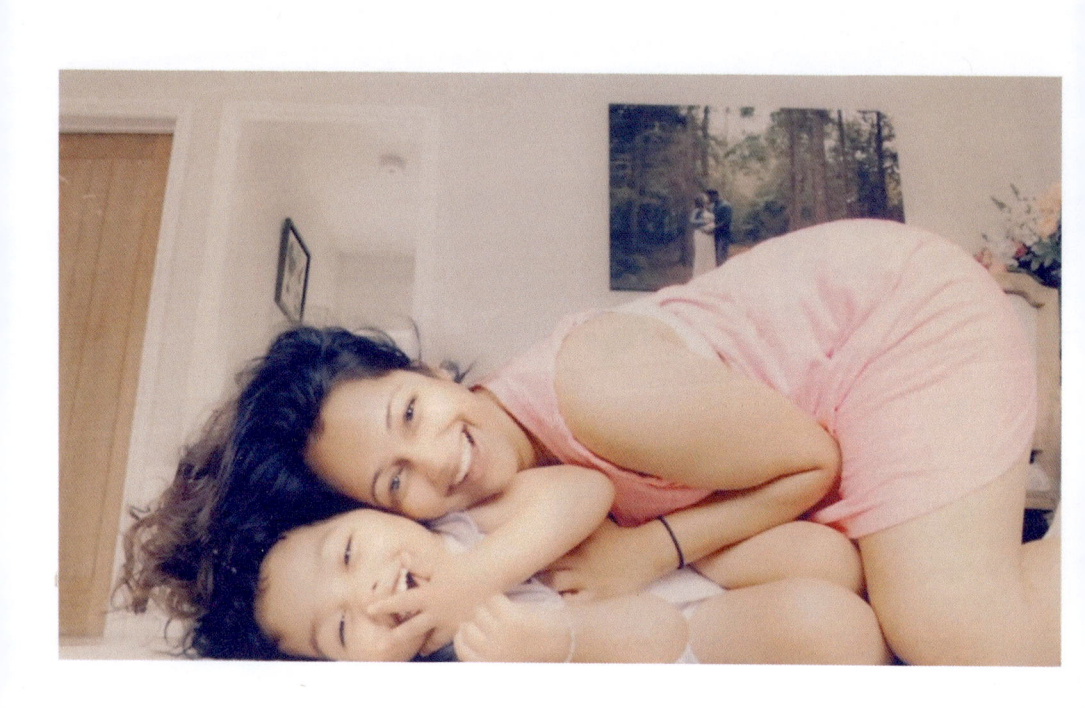

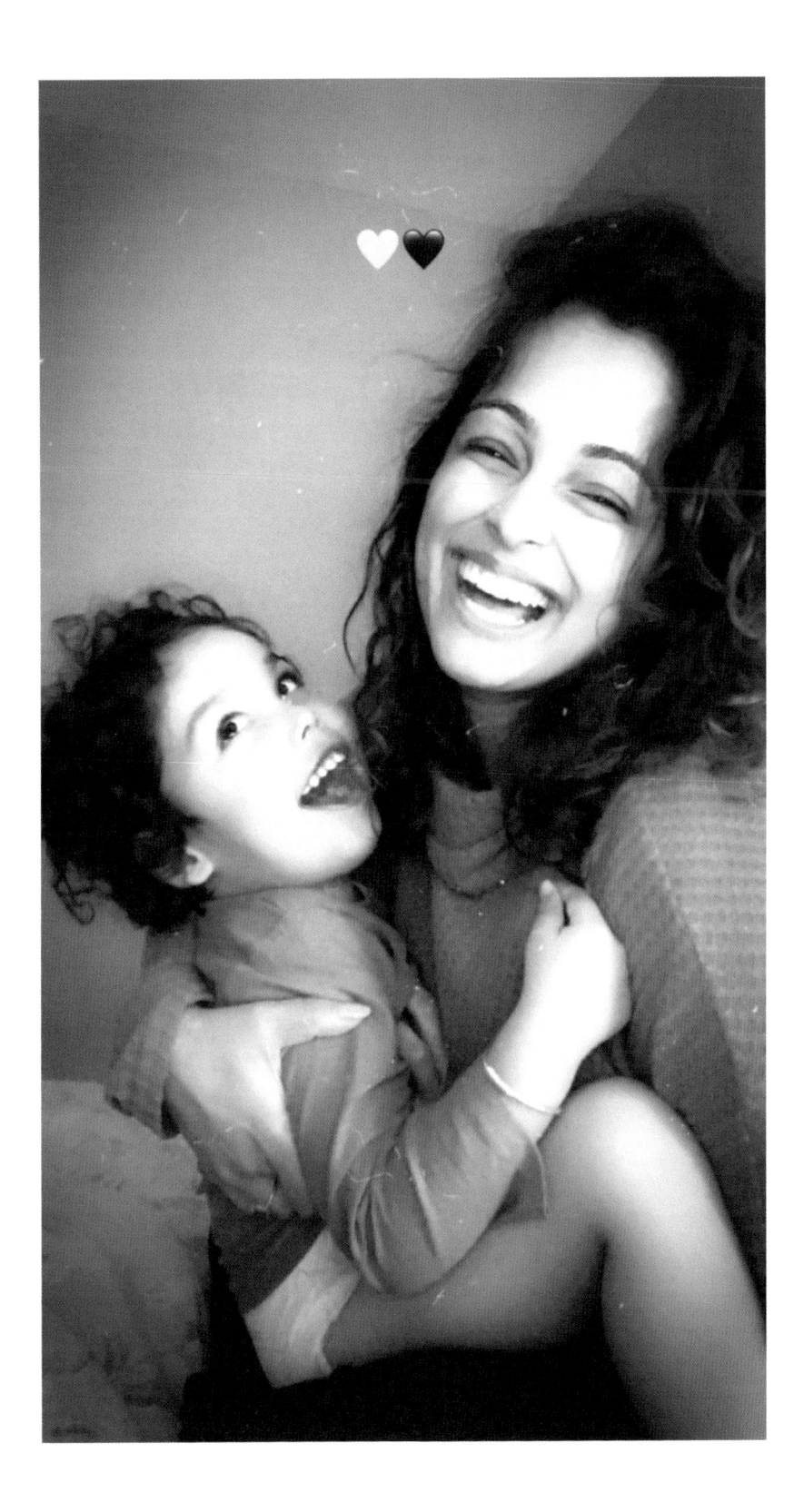

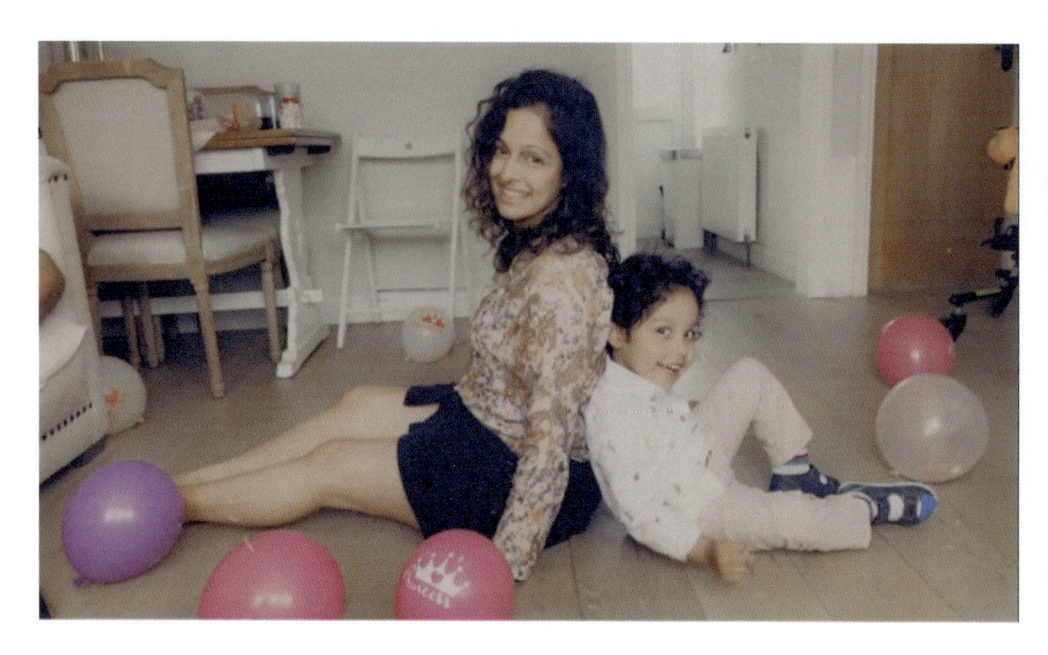

I'll have your back forever Rèyan

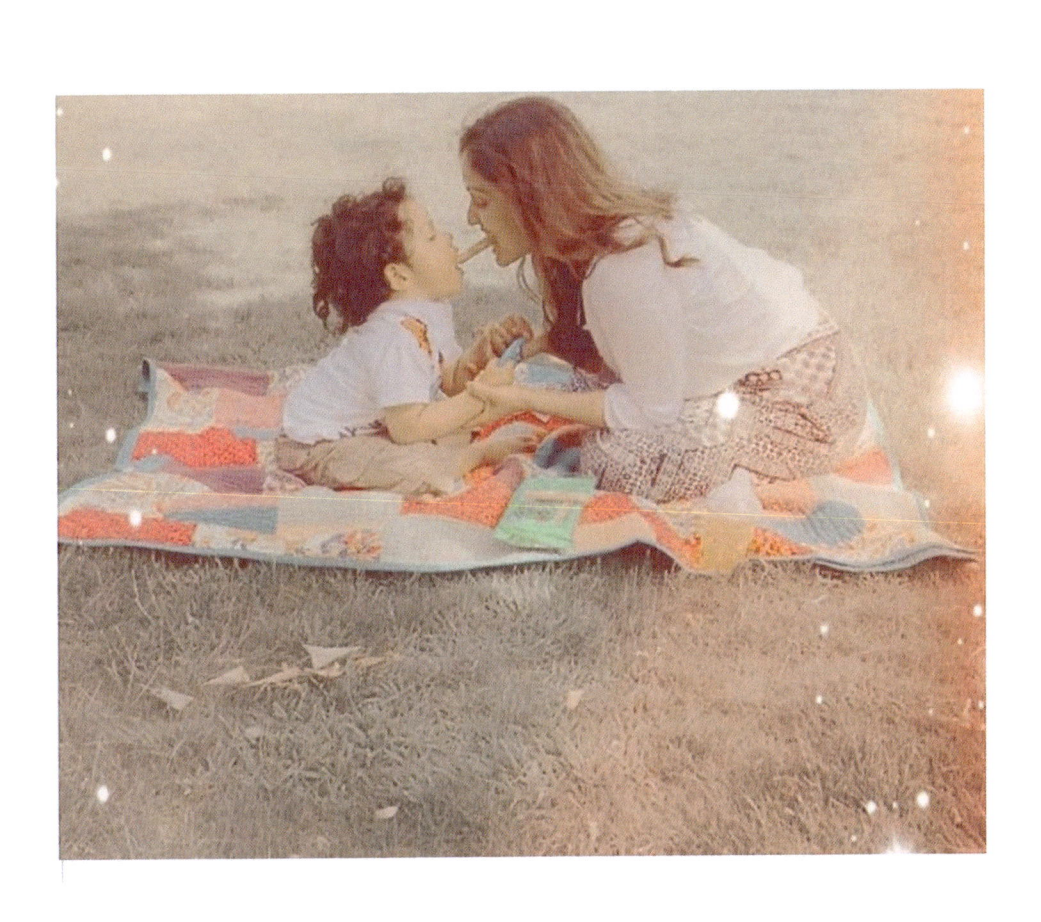

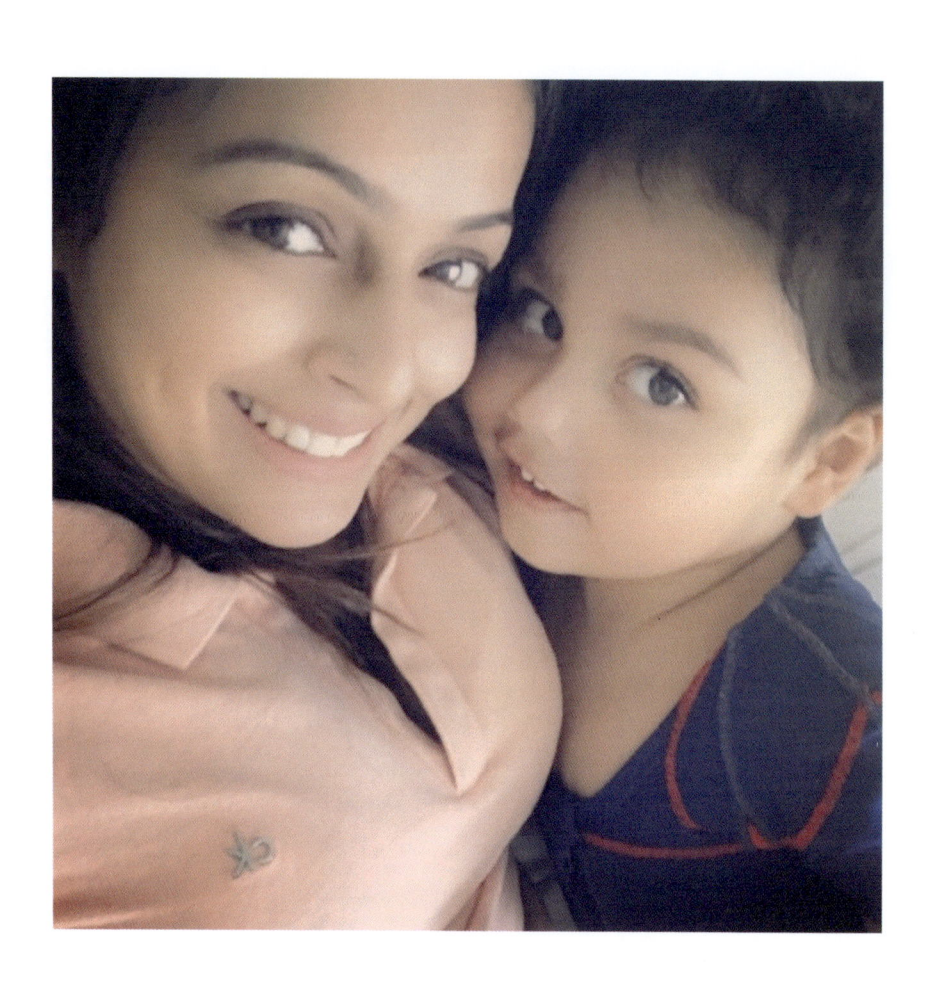

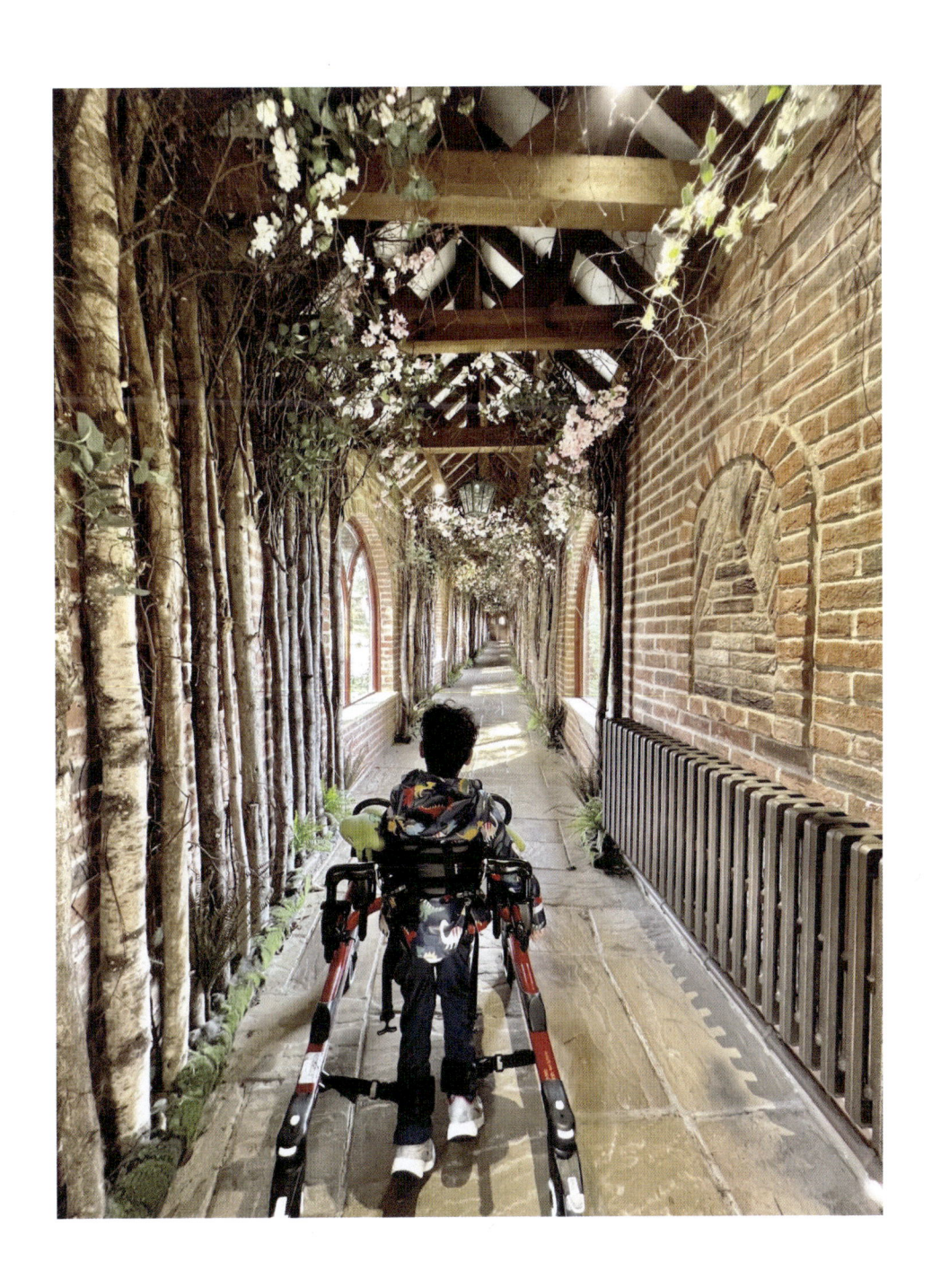

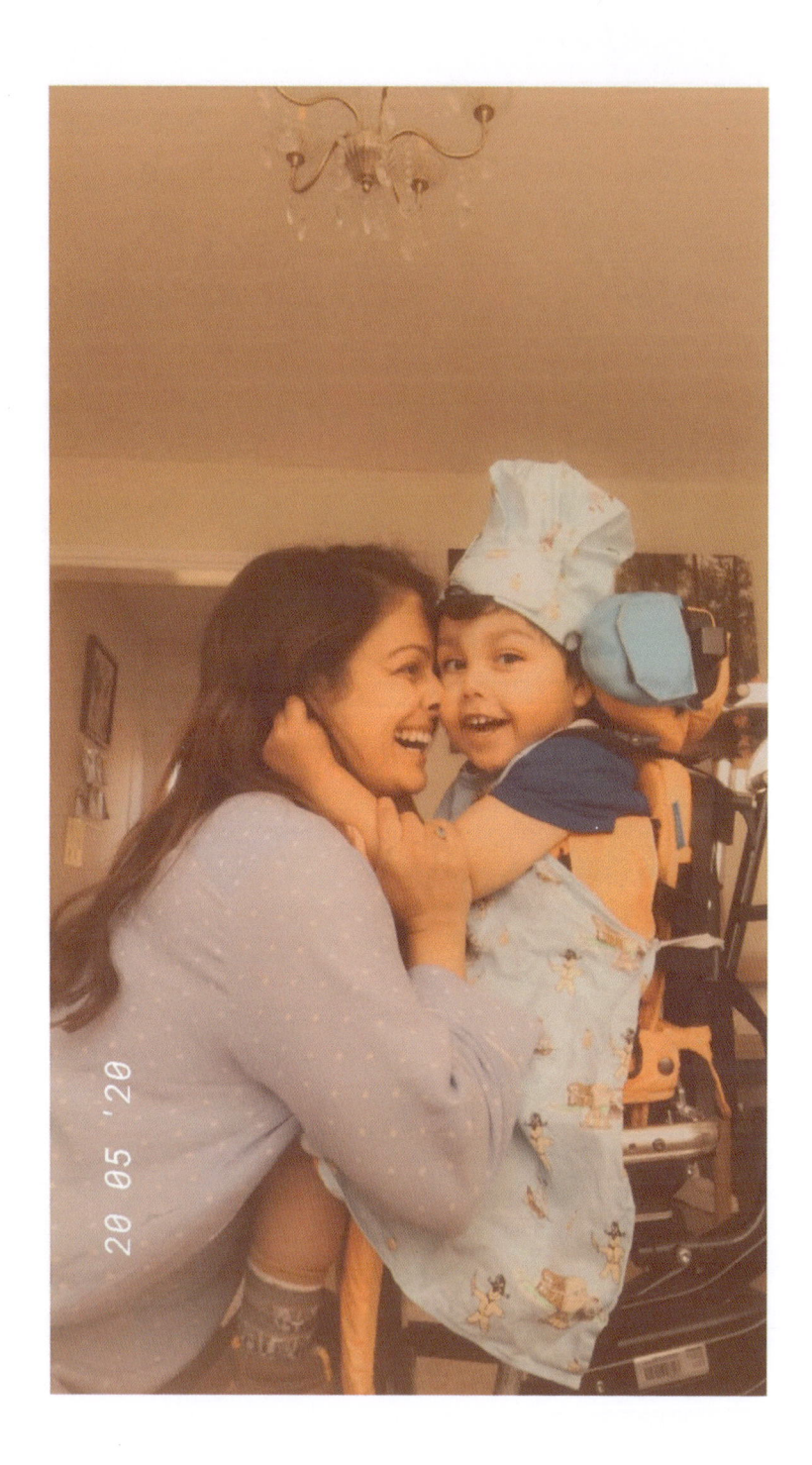

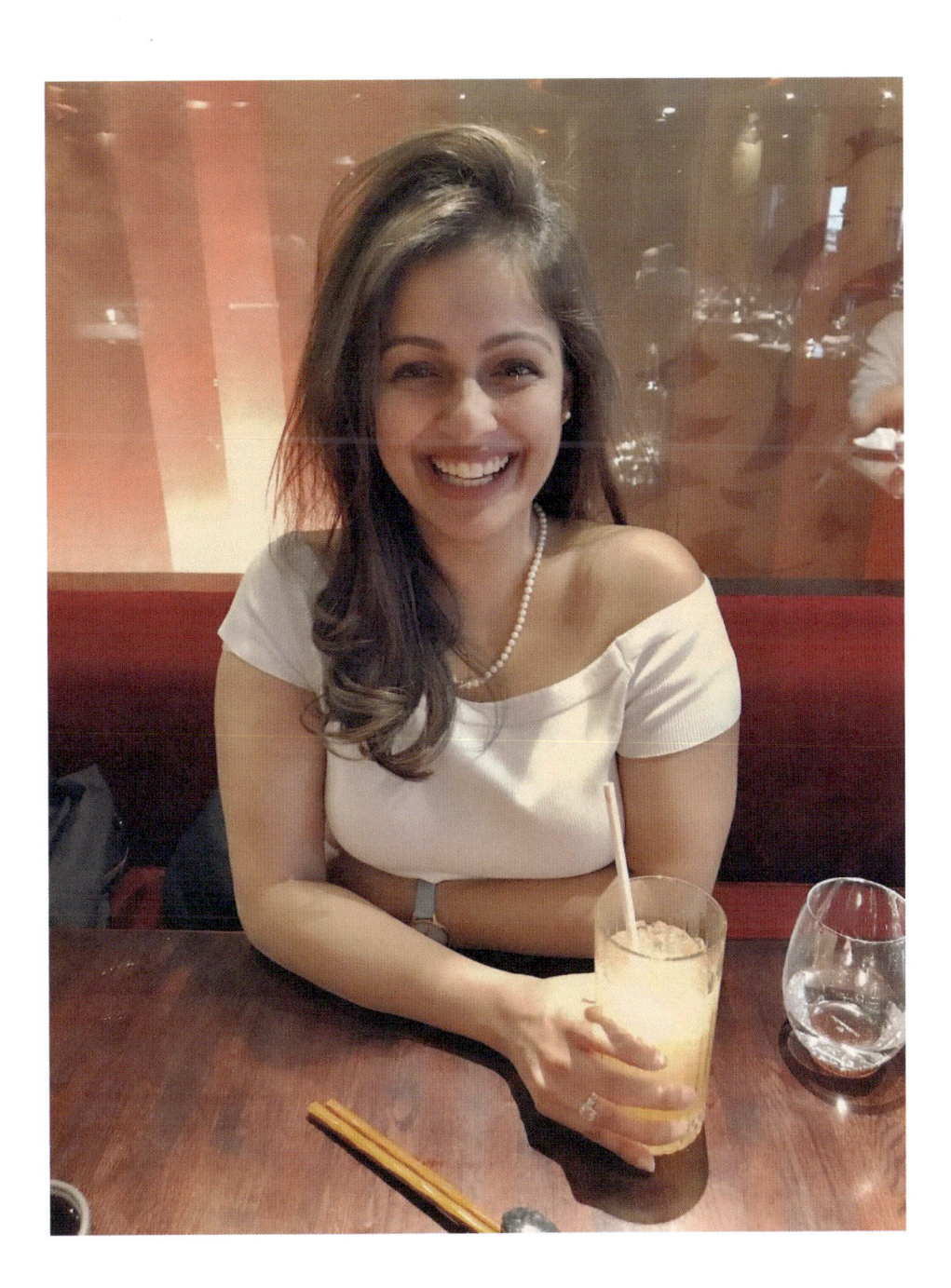

StoryTerrace